BREAKING THE AGING CODE

MAXIMIZING YOUR DNA FUNCTION FOR OPTIMAL HEALTH AND LONGEVITY

VINCENT C. GIAMPAPA, M.D., F.A.C.S.,
AND MIRYAM EHRLICH WILLIAMSON

T0273567

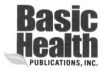

Basic
Health
PUBLICATIONS, INC.

The information contained in this book is based upon the research and personal and pro-fessional experiences of the author. It is not intended as a substitute for consulting with your physician or other healthcare provider. Any attempt to diagnose and treat an illness should be done under the direction of a healthcare professional.

The publisher does not advocate the use of any particular healthcare protocol but believes the information in this book should be available to the public. The publisher and author are not responsible for any adverse effects or consequences resulting from the use of the sug-gestions, preparations, or procedures discussed in this book. Should the reader have any questions concerning the appropriateness of any procedures or preparation mentioned, the author and the publisher strongly suggest consulting a professional healthcare advisor.

BASIC HEALTH PUBLICATIONS, INC.
8200 Boulevard East
North Bergen, NJ 07047
1-201-868-8336

Library of Congress Cataloging-in-Publication Data
Giampapa, Vincent C.
    Breaking the aging code : maximizing your DNA function
for optimal health and longevity / Vincent C. Giampapa and
Miryam Ehrlich Williamson.
        p. cm.
Includes bibliographical references and index.
    ISBN 1-59120-079-2
    1. Aging—Physiological aspects. 2. DNA. 3. Longevity. 4. Health.
I. Williamson, Miryam Ehrlich. II. Title.
    QP86.G465   2003
    613—dc22

                                    2003021363

Editor: Susan E. Davis
Typesetter/Book design: Gary A. Rosenberg
Cover design: Mike Stromberg

Printed in the United States of America

10   9   8   7   6   5   4   3   2   1

Contents

To Susan,
who keeps me anchored.

—V.C.G.

To Ed,
who puts the wind in my sails.

—M.E.W.

Acknowledgments

For the past decade I have had the pleasure and honor to share new ideas and concepts about how we age with an extraordinary group of human beings. This book is dedicated to these special physicians and pioneers who have had the courage and vision to conceive of a new medical society and a new medical paradigm. They changed how we view the aging process and unshackled our minds from the constraints of medical dogma that existed for hundreds of years.

This special group has changed the quality and quantity of life for our present generation, as well as for generations to come. We will all benefit from their refusal to accept the limits of contemporary medical minds as the limits of reality.

I express my deepest thanks to Eric Braverman, M.D.; Stanley Burzynski, M.D., Ph.D.; Ward Dean, M.D.; Bob Goldman, M.D.; Thierry Hertoge, M.D.; Steven M. Hedfflin, M.D.; Dharma Khalsa, M.D.; Ron Klatz, M.D.; Steve Novell, M.D.; Chong Park, M.D.; Nicholas V. Perricone, M.D.; Ronald Pero, Ph.D.; Oscar M. Ramirez, M.D.; Steven Sinatra, M.D.; James Smith, M.D.; and Aristo Vojdani, Ph.D.

—Vincent C. Giampapa, M.D.

Special thanks to Susan E. Davis, a superb developmental editor and project manager, for her exceptional organizational skills and dedication to perfection.

—Vincent C. Giampapa, M.D.
—Miryam Ehrlich Williamson

Introduction

KEEP YOUR MIND OPEN TO CHANGE ALL THE TIME. WELCOME IT.
COURT IT. IT IS ONLY BY EXAMINING AND REEXAMINING YOUR
OPINIONS AND IDEAS THAT YOU CAN PROGRESS.
—*Dale Carnegie*

The rate at which we age is governed by a complex of variable factors over which, until recently, we thought we had little chance of exercising control. Now that science has taken the giant step of mapping the human genome, the genetic material that makes human beings simultaneously alike and unique, we have the potential to control more of our individual destinies than past generations dared to dream.

The first decade of the twenty-first century is an exciting time. Scientists are adding to the understanding of our genetic blueprint on an almost daily basis. As we learn each new fact, we reach a deeper knowledge of why and how we age. Our knowledge base of techniques to retard the aging process is doubling every two years. Since 1990 we have accumulated more information on aging than was obtained over the previous 2,000 years. What was once as arcane as alchemy has become molecular biology; what was considered magic is now quantum physics and genetics.

We have also just begun to understand the critical impact of our environment—the air we breathe, the water we drink, what and how we eat, our internal flora and fauna, our psychological makeup, and the social milieu in which we live and work—on our health and longevity, and more

1

specifically, on our genes. Genetic damage, not the genes we inherited, dictates why most people around the world have a life span of sixty to seventy years. The prevalence of genetic damage in most people is the reason it is so remarkable that anyone lives to be 100 years old. It is so unusual that by tradition the President of the United States sends a letter of congratulations to every citizen who reaches that landmark of age.

We do not need to assume that illness is inevitable as we grow older or accept damage to our genes as unavoidable. In this book you will find information that will change your assumptions about aging, guidance to help you overcome the negative perception that to be old means to be sick, and the means to control and retard the process of your own aging.

In June 2000, researchers from the United States and Britain announced that they had deciphered the human genome, the sequence of chemical "letters" containing the basic instructions for building and running the human body. This 3-billion-letter code contains the genetic makeup of all human beings. To the surprise of those who mapped the human genome, what was originally thought to be a collection of about 100,000 genes turned out to be approximately 30,000, only a few thousand (perhaps 10 percent) of which are active at any time during our lives. We now know that the set of active genes changes as we grow, mature, and age. We used to think that each gene bore the code for a single purpose, but it now has become evident that each may play multiple roles.

DECIPHERING THE CODE...

Most of the body's 100 trillion CELLS contain a NUCLEUS with 46 CHROMOSOMES, each one made of a long, coiled-up strand of DNA. Thousands of sections along every strand represent GENES, which are coded instructions for making the proteins needed to construct a complete human organism.

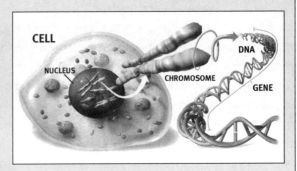

Our bodies are made up of some 100 trillion cells, differentiated according to the work they perform. The single most important breakthrough that led to the mapping of the human genome was the discovery of DNA in the nucleus of each of these cells. Even though 99.9 percent of the DNA found in the human body is identical from person to person, DNA also contains the genetic code that makes each of us unique. It is that remaining 0.1 percent that differentiates each of us from everyone else.

Environmental factors can cause stress and damage to DNA, changing the way genes function within our bodies. Hostile environments can give rise to malfunctioning genes and, ultimately, cause aging, disease, and death. If DNA carries our genetic code, then a subset of DNA carries the code that determines how we age, and it can be negatively affected by environmental factors. It is to breaking this code—learning to understand and manage it—that this book is dedicated.

Science is already beginning to use our rudimentary understanding of the genetic code to perform gene therapy to treat a limited number of diseases. Eventually, although perhaps not for several decades, we will be able to use information about specific genes to intercede in the aging process. But we know enough about the aging code now to make a difference in how we age, to improve our health and increase longevity.

This book suggests a new way of looking at how we age. It offers a model that you can incorporate into your lifestyle to achieve a longer life than would otherwise be possible, as well as a better quality of life as you age. The premise of this book is the radical concept that *we are built for self-repair, and are not programmed to die.* Contrary to conventional wisdom, which holds that we die once our cells have divided and reproduced themselves a set number of times, information now seems to indicate that the capacity for cell division is not as restricted as we thought. This means that we have the potential to live longer, healthier lives, under the right circumstances and in the right environment.

Central to this new paradigm of aging is the belief that we can limit damage to DNA and repair what harm is done, allowing us to maximize our genetic potential. To do this requires that we control the four main cellular processes—glycation, inflammation, oxidation, and methylation—that take place within each cell and influence the age-related changes that every body undergoes. Taken together, these processes can be viewed as an equation we can use to break the "aging code" stored in our genes. Success with this endeavor will forestall the diseases we associate with aging and slow the changes to our appearance that occur with the passage of time.

Developing an anti-aging regimen has obvious benefits for us individually, but it also will benefit our economy and society as a whole. By 1995, the most recent year for which such data are available, members of the baby boom generation (the 77 million people born between 1947 and 1964) had collectively saved 15 trillion dollars for their retirement (some of which surely disappeared during the recession that began in 2001). But if current disease patterns of aging continue unabated, this generation will require 184 trillion dollars to maintain their health as they age. There is not that much money on the entire planet.

Experts anticipated that 14 percent of the United States budget would be spent on geriatric medicine in 2003. If the health span—that is, maintaining oneself in a healthy, productive condition—of every American could be extended by only one year, the United States economy would save 1 trillion to 3 trillion dollars in healthcare costs and lost productivity. If prevailing disease patterns continue through the next twenty years, the healthcare system of the United States will become bankrupt. Current medical anti-aging technology can provide a healthy life expectancy of 90 to 100 years to at least half of today's 76 million baby boomers.

In summary, our age-management goals are to control the negative effects of the twenty-first century environment we live in; to manage the processes that lead to aging; and to boost the ratio of DNA repair to DNA damage, resulting in less cell mutation and more accurate cell copies during cell replication. This book will tell you how you can accomplish this. You may need professional medical help for some of it, but you can do most of it yourself.

CHAPTER 1

Aging: Processes and Theories

MAN'S MIND STRETCHED TO A NEW IDEA,
NEVER GOES BACK TO ITS ORIGINAL DIMENSION.
—*Oliver Wendell Holmes*

Any successful attempt to minimize the damage commonly associated with aging requires understanding and control of the processes that take place at the cellular level. These seven fundamental processes affect genetic expression, the process by which genes are activated and suppressed, and are interrelated, with each one having a direct impact on the others. Taken together they form the basis of a new way to look at aging and find ways to retard its harmful effects. Understanding these processes allows us to discover ways to intervene and prevent damage, starting at the intimate level of DNA within the cell and moving on to control of hormones and other chemical messengers. We can also address environmental variables, both within and outside of our bodies.

THE SEVEN PROCESSES

Each of the following seven processes will be explained more fully later in the book. For now, some basic knowledge will enable you to understand the theories of aging on which we base our anti-aging management program.

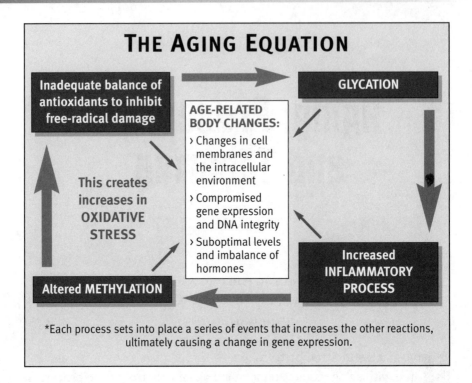

THE AGING EQUATION

Inadequate balance of antioxidants to inhibit free-radical damage

GLYCATION

AGE-RELATED BODY CHANGES:
› Changes in cell membranes and the intracellular environment
› Compromised gene expression and DNA integrity
› Suboptimal levels and imbalance of hormones

This creates increases in OXIDATIVE STRESS

Altered METHYLATION

Increased INFLAMMATORY PROCESS

*Each process sets into place a series of events that increases the other reactions, ultimately causing a change in gene expression.

Glycation

Carbohydrates and a small fraction of proteins turn into glucose (a sugar) when we digest them. Insulin is the instrument by which our cells store glucose for energy. As we age, our cells become less sensitive to insulin, leaving more glucose in the bloodstream. Type 2 (insulin resistant) diabetes is the best-known result of insulin insensitivity. Its chief characteristic is an abnormally high level of glucose in the blood. Many people have undiagnosed diabetes, or a prediabetic condition in which blood sugar levels are higher than optimal, but not high enough to meet the criterion for outright diabetes. These people, as well as those diagnosed with diabetes, are particularly subject to glycation.

Glycation is the process in which extra glucose molecules attach themselves to proteins, altering the proteins' structure and function, and rendering them unable to perform as they should. This attachment, termed *cross-linkage,* is the basis for one theory of aging.

Inflammation

Under normal circumstances, the inflammation response reflects the body's effort to heal itself from injury or infection. Capillaries, the smallest blood vessels, dilate in the affected area and bring additional blood supply and immune system cells to the site to penetrate the affected tissues and carry out the healing process. Once the injury has healed or the infection has cleared up, pain and swelling subside and the tissues return to their normal state. This process describes *acute inflammation.* It occurs in response to a number of specific triggers and ends when the condition is resolved.

Chronic inflammation is quite another matter. Generally, a condition is considered chronic when it has persisted for three months or longer. Chronic inflammation results when the immune system mistakenly identifies some cells as foreign invaders and sets about destroying them. This misdirected attempt at self-healing is called the *autoimmune response.* Rheumatoid arthritis, multiple sclerosis, and Type 1 (insulin dependent) diabetes are examples of autoimmune diseases. Such diseases are just as likely to attack the young and middle-aged as the elderly, and are not necessarily associated with aging.

But another kind of chronic inflammation is brought about by excessive quantities of certain hormonelike substances known as *eicosanoids,* and by immune system cells known as *cytokines,* both of which increase with age. Both cytokines and eicosanoids perform beneficial functions when they are present in the proper proportions and cause trouble only when they get out of control. Among other ailments, chronic inflammation can damage cells lining the joints, causing osteoarthritis; it can harm brain cells, causing dementia; and it can attack arterial walls and heart valves, leading to heart attack and stroke. The *Autoimmune Theory of Aging* refers to the effects of chronic inflammation.

Free Radicals and Oxidative Stress

As essential as it is for life, oxygen can be a stress factor for the body because it is subject to chemical alteration when exposed to environmental toxins, including air pollution, tobacco smoke, chemicals in our food and water, radiation (as in sunlight), and certain biochemical reactions. Fortunately, our bodies are well equipped to cope with this oxidative burden. But as we age, our ability to fight off the effects of oxidation declines. One visible sign of this phenomenon is *lipofuscin,* more commonly known as "age spots." They signal an accumulation of oxidized fatty acids and other cellular "garbage" that the body has been unable to clear and that accumulate in the skin.

Oxidative stress that is not successfully dealt with by the body results in the formation of free radicals. These are highly charged atoms and molecules that are missing one electron, making them chemically unstable. Since seeking stability is the prime directive of every atom and molecule, free radicals attempt to steal electrons from other molecules in our cells, creating more free radicals in a chain reaction as they scramble to replace their missing electrons. It has been estimated that each of our cells undergoes 10,000 free-radical hits per day. Unchecked oxidative stress can damage the DNA that carries our genetic code, with serious and possibly devastating effects on our health. The *Free-Radical Theory of Aging* details this process.

Faulty Gene Expression

Most of our genes are active during the embryonic stage of development. Throughout life, genes are switched on and off, determining which proteins should be manufactured and thus how cells should develop and function. Genes are activated when a new developmental stage is reached and become blocked when their expression is no longer needed. An example we have all experienced is the activation during puberty of genes that govern the production of sex hormones and secondary sex characteristics such as the growth of the testes in adolescent boys, breasts in adolescent girls, and pubic hair in both sexes. Eventually, we will all experience the deactivation of these same genes as we near the end of middle age.

Several mechanisms provide for the expression and suppression of genes. One such mechanism is *methylation,* in which a molecule called a *methyl group,* consisting of one carbon atom and three hydrogen atoms, attaches itself to a specific portion of the DNA. This is the signal that a particular gene is not necessary for the cell's function and should not be expressed. Methylation is crucial to life: it provides for the specialization of cells. Although all of our cells contain the same genetic information, the activation of some genes and suppression of others is what gives each cell its specific function. Different genes are activated in a skin cell than are activated in a cell in the intestinal lining, for example. Without methylation, all genes would be expressed at once, instead of according to the normal schedule of human development and cell specialization.

Evidence emerging from recent research suggests that brain aging and, possibly, cancer and cardiac aging are, in part, consequences of faulty methylation patterns. The *Methylation Control of Gene Activation and Silencing Theory* holds that the progressive silencing of genes is a major factor in aging and, ultimately, death. The theory holds that other molecular switches or naturally occurring compounds can reactivate genes that can provide a number of anti-aging benefits.

Cell Membrane Abnormalities

Each of the body's trillions of cells is surrounded by a membrane that separates it from its neighbors. The structure of the cell membrane makes it selectively permeable so only certain substances are allowed to enter and leave. The cell takes in nutrients and disposes of the waste products of normal cell metabolism through this membrane.

Free-radical damage can severely disrupt the structure of the cell membrane, impairing its ability to regulate the passage of nutrients and waste products into and out of the cell. Over time toxins and metabolic waste products accumulate, changing the delicate balance of substances such as water, salts, fats, carbohydrates, and proteins within the cell. Additionally, because healthy cell membranes are essential to effective nervous system function, oxidation of the cell membrane can impair cell-to-cell communication and the transmission of nerve impulses. If the membranes of cells important to immune function are damaged, the body's defense system becomes less efficient, and the immune reaction to invading viruses and bacteria becomes slowed. Free radicals can also wreak havoc on the parts of cells that control cellular metabolism, thus impairing the cell's ability to produce energy necessary to survival.

Changes in acidity and hydration occur within cells whose membranes have been compromised. This leads to an insufficient supply of repair building blocks and less than optimal creation of new proteins. This in turn leads to the accumulation of damaged protein compounds in our "cellular soup," both inside and outside the cells. The *Membrane Hypothesis of Aging* accounts for these effects, and explains the visible results of aging seen in the skin.

Hormonal Imbalances

Hormones are our body's chemical messengers. They are secreted by specific glands and travel in the blood to the places where they do their work, affecting all aspects of body function including growth and development, tissue repair and regeneration, metabolism, reproduction, and even mood. Some of the more familiar hormones are insulin, glucagon, cortisol, growth hormone, thyroid hormones, estrogen, and testosterone.

The hypothalamus is the part of the brain that receives messages from nerves about the internal condition of the body and the external environment. It responds to this information by sending signals to the appropriate glands to release hormones. Once hormones are released into the bloodstream they travel to particular target cells to deliver their chemical messages and cause a specific biological response. Ideally, our hormones exist in a delicate balance and deliver their messages to the cells accurately and reliably. But hormone imbalances become increasingly common with advancing age. For example, cells may resist the signal of the hormone insulin, causing the pancreas to overwork, secreting ever more insulin. An excess of insulin causes a cascade of effects on other hormones, and some become elevated while others become depressed. Many hormone imbalances can be corrected nutritionally if they are detected early enough, but some may require medication.

The link between hormonal imbalance and the aging process is well known. Levels of certain hormones, such as estrogen, testosterone, and human growth hormone, decline with age. In other instances, the body becomes less responsive to hormonal action as it does with insulin, the secretion of which increases in response. Age-related problems that have been linked to hormonal imbalances include depression, osteoporosis, heart disease, and sexual dysfunction.

Compromised DNA Structural Integrity

Throughout life, our DNA is subject to the damaging effects of free radicals, the result both of normal cell metabolism and of environmental assaults coming from outside the body. DNA errors accumulate and are passed on to newly replicated cells, in much the same way that a faulty photocopy of an original document passes on its errors to future generations of photocopies. The result of these errors is faulty production of proteins and enzymes, impairing the cellular machinery within each of the 100 trillion cells that make up the human body. Damaged gene replication also causes deficiencies in the reserves of undifferentiated stem cells within all of the organ systems. Stem cells are capable of taking on the characteristics of cells in whatever part of the body they are needed. Since they can be used anywhere in the body, an adequate stem cell reserve is essential to maintaining optimal organ health and function.

Because healthy DNA is essential to health and longevity, the body has mechanisms for repairing DNA damage to maintain the integrity of the genetic code. Enzymes and other proteins identify damaged DNA, then remove and replace injured segments of the deficient strand. However, as we age, DNA repair becomes less effective. Ultimately, repair mechanisms cannot keep pace with the rate of damage. The result is an added burden from copies of damaged cells. When copies of cells become genetically "unreadable" the cells age and die instead of continuing to replicate.

Even a small (5 to 15 percent) reduction in DNA damage and improvement in DNA repair can yield remarkable results in terms of slowing the aging process and improving quality of life. Before we begin our attempt to alter these fundamental processes, a review of past and present aging theories will lead us to a deeper understanding of age management and anti-aging therapies.

THEORIES OF AGING

The desire to explain phenomena that we observe is a characteristic of human nature. People have always made up stories, many of which evolved into myths, to explain the existence of a sky full of stars; how mountains and oceans came into being; and other natural occurrences such as eclipses, earthquakes, and floods. All of scientific endeavor is an attempt to find explanations, so it is no surprise that theories to unravel the mysteries associated with birth, aging, and death abound.

The existence of a large number of theories regarding aging reflects the fact that, in reality, aging has no single cause. It is a complex series of events that take place over the years as each of us interacts with the environment. Different theories emphasize different processes and events; none is wholly correct or incorrect. Each theory is like a piece in a jigsaw puzzle. Until recently, attempts to assemble the puzzle led to the realization that some of the pieces were missing. Now, with the discovery of DNA and the mapping of the human genome, it is possible to construct a theory that synthesizes past theories, adds our current understanding of the role of DNA in aging, and factors in the importance of stem cells, so that we emerge with a new paradigm of aging. It is on this new paradigm, detailed at the end of this chapter, that we base our anti-aging activities.

Early Theories

In the 1940s, scientists interested in the role of gene mutation in aging observed that radiation not only increased genetic mutation in animals, but also accelerated the rate at which they aged. Not long after this came the discovery of *cross-linkage*, in which glucose molecules link to proteins, obstructing the passage of nutrients and waste products between cells and causing damage to genes. This theory has led current-day anti-aging researchers to focus on the importance of glycation.

Scientists involved in anti-aging research discovered early on that environmental factors were implicated in cell damage. *The Wear-and-Tear Theory* of aging focuses on the proposition that the body and its cells are damaged by overuse and abuse: that specific organs are worn down by toxins in the diet and in the environment. This theory concentrates in particular on the consumption of fat, sugar, caffeine, and alcohol, as well as the harmful effects of the sun's ultraviolet rays. It is one of the precursors of more sophisticated theories on wear and tear at the cellular level, including the *Waste Accumulation Theory*, which proposes that cells produce more waste than they can properly dispose of, including toxins that accumulate and ultimately kill cells by interfering with their normal functions.

The *Neuroendocrine Theory* elaborated on theories of wear and tear by focusing specifically on the neuroendocrine (glandular) system. This theory suggests that hormones are vital for repairing and regulating body functions. When aging causes a decrease in production of any of the endocrine hormones, it alters the body's ability to repair and regulate itself. In essence, the neuroendocrine system is likened to a symphony orchestra, in which discord from any one instrument ruins the entire performance. Because of this theory, hormone replacement is a key component in any anti-aging program.

Some early theories propose a kind of *genetic determinism* in which each individual inherits the genes for certain age-related diseases, and these genes determine how quickly a person ages and how long he or she lives. Although many aspects of genetic determinism have been supported by research on DNA, the notion that the genes we inherit completely control our destiny has been replaced by the understanding that we inherit genetic *tendencies,* not genetic *certainties.* We therefore have significant potential to improve both how we age and the quality of our lives as we age.

Finally, two theories dealing with immune function have contributed to our current understanding of the aging process. The *Thymic Stimulating Theory* identifies the thymus gland as the master gland controlling immune function. The thymus gland is at its largest at birth and continues to shrink until death. Studies have shown that thymic secretions are helpful in restoring poorly functioning immune systems in people of all ages. Thymic hormones probably play a role in controlling the production of hormones that affect brain function, which in turn affects the central pacemakers of aging. The complementary *Autoimmune Theory* says that as the body ages, its ability to fight certain diseases declines. In a sense, the immune system becomes self-destructive, reacting against its own proteins. This theory gains credibility in view of the effects of aging on the gastrointestinal tract and the prevalence of *leaky gut syndrome,* which has been seen to be directly related to autoimmunity as people age.

Each of the preceding theories contribute to our current understanding of how we age. Other more recent theories take us even further.

Free-Radical Theory

A free radical is an atom or molecule that has an uneven number of electrons. Ordinarily, electrons exist in pairs, with one positive and one negative charge, so that they neutralize each other. Atoms and molecules with a neutral charge are chemically stable. When an atom loses an electron, it becomes unstable. In its quest for equilibrium, it breaks the electron bonds in nearby molecules to steal an electron. Although it neutralizes itself, more free radicals are created and a chain reaction is started as each affected atom or molecule tries to restabilize itself by stealing another electron.

This process is known as oxidation. Under ideal circumstances, our bodies are well equipped to deal with oxidation. Few people, however, live in ideal circumstances. Environmental toxins exacerbate the oxidative process, leading to *oxidative stress,* which, in turn, damages cell membranes and genetic material and causes a host of age-related diseases including heart disease and dementia.

The creation of free radicals is a byproduct of the metabolic process that creates energy in our cells. Without oxidation, the body would be unable to produce energy, maintain immunity, use hormones, or even contract muscles. Cell metabolism requires the existence of unbalanced electrons to provide electrical energy. As is so often true in nature, a beneficial process has its detrimental side. Without oxidation there would be no life, but because of it our cells and genes are subject to damage.

Oxidation begins at birth and continues throughout life. Early in life, its effects are relatively minor because the body has extensive repair and replacement mechanisms in place that allow the cells and organs to work optimally. Over time, however, the cumulative effects of free-radical damage begin to take their toll. The most obvious physical manifestation of free-radical damage appears in the form of facial wrinkles, caused by damage to collagen and elastin, which keep skin smooth, moist, flexible and elastic. This is why people who smoke tobacco, one of the toxic substances most responsible for oxidative stress, usually have deep wrinkles on their faces. In addition to damaging cell membranes, free radicals can cause defects in DNA, the bearer of the genetic code, leading to faulty copies during cell reproduction and impeding the creation of proteins, enzymes, and hormones.

Membrane Hypothesis of Aging

A recent blending of the Waste Accumulation and Free-Radical theories is the hypothesis that by damaging the cell membrane, free radicals render the membrane unable to let nutrients in and waste products out. As waste products build up within the cell, the cell becomes dehydrated. This interferes with the normal flow of electrolytes into and out of the cell, causing toxins and the cell's metabolic wastes to accumulate and eventually bringing about the death of the cell.

Hayflick Limit Theory

Named for Dr. Leonard Hayflick, the cell biologist who developed it, this theory is one of the most important contributions to the study of aging. It suggests that the aging process is controlled by a biological clock contained within each living cell. Dr. Hayflick studied human fibroblast cells from the lung, skin, muscle, and heart and found them to have a limited life span; they divided approximately fifty times over a period of years and then suddenly stopped. Nutrition seemed to have an effect on the frequency of cell divisions. Overfed cells made up to fifty divisions in a year, but underfed cells took up to three times as long to make the same number of divisions. This information has been used as the basis of research on the relationship between caloric restriction and life extension.

Mitochondria Theory of Aging

Mitochondria are energy-producing organelles—tiny organs within cells—that produce adenosine triphosphate (ATP), the primary source of cellular energy. ATP fuels the nuclear and mitochondrial genetic machinery to allow cell reproduction to occur. Not only do mitochondria produce energy, but they also produce vast amounts of potentially damaging free radicals. Mitochondria have limited DNA repair mechanisms, and thus are an extremely sensitive target for free-radical damage. This theory builds on the free-radical theory in asserting that free radicals directly damage mitochondrial DNA. This is the basic reason to introduce age-management programs to people as young as in their thirties.

Telomerase Theory of Aging

Recent research in genetic engineering has identified a structure called a *telomere* that appears to have a significant influence over cell division and cell death. Chromosomes, the structures that hold our genetic information, are arranged in the form of an X, so that each chromosome has four arms. Fitting over the end of each arm is a sheathlike telomere. Telomeres maintain the integrity of chromosomes during cell division. Every time a cell divides, its telomeres become shorter. As the telomere shortens, it exposes other genes, which become active and start producing proteins. When telomeres become so short that they are only at the end of the chromosome's arm, they signal the cell to stop dividing and die. Thus, this theory identifies telomeres as a kind of biological clock that limits the life of each cell to a preset number of divisions. Since cell division is essential to life itself, as the number of cells that fail to divide increases, organ health declines and eventually death occurs.

Scientists have discovered an enzyme they call *telomerase*, found only in germ cells, cancer cells, and stem cells, that can lengthen telemeres by repairing and replacing them. Research now focuses on the possibility of finding a substance that stimulates the creation of telomerase, thereby increasing the number of times a cell can divide, delaying cell death and in effect turning back the hands on the biological clock.

New research reveals that even people in their nineties have telomeres that are not at the end of their chromosomes, suggesting that we have the potential to live longer than has been previously assumed. This theory shows how important it is to focus on decreasing damage and improving repair to our DNA.

Methylation Control of Gene Activation and Silencing Theory

According to this theory, most genes are active during the development of an embryo, but are silenced by methylation at birth. Some are reactivated at a later time and others are suppressed throughout life. Adult cells have an established methylation pattern in their DNA that is an essential component of the aging process. After age twenty-five, increasing numbers of genes are silenced as life progresses. This silencing process is a major factor leading to progressive aging and ultimately death. In addition, if the silencing affects tumor-suppressor genes for any reason, the aging person may develop cancer.

Several natural substances have been identified that can reactivate tumor-suppressor genes in cancer patients. These substances, discovered by Dr. Stanley Burzynski in Houston, Texas, act as molecular switches and can also reactivate genes involved in some aspects of aging. The term for these molecular switches is *antineoplastons*. While activating tumor-suppressor genes to help alleviate the potential cancer, antineoplastons also turn on other genes, which can provide aging patients with a number of benefits. According to this theory, we may be able to stop and even reverse the established adult pattern of methylation with properly designed antineoplastons that deactivate certain genes and activate more youthful ones.

Unified DNA Damage Theory of Aging (UDDTA)

Clearly, there is no lack of concepts and theories to explain why we all eventually grow old and die. As is true in all science, many theories overlap and complement one another. Just as clearly, there is no single cause of aging. How it proceeds depends on a combination of genetic inheritance, environmental factors, and the oxidative process. The rest of this book addresses a new theory that synthesizes those that have been proposed previously, and also provides a program of lifestyle changes designed to capitalize on what we now know about the aging process and how to control it.

According to this new theory, human beings are not irreversibly programmed to age and die, as is currently thought, but are programmed for self-repair and longevity. Although we inherited a unique genetic code from our ancestors, including the part that determines how we age, we can modify our aging code by attending to our body's ability to repair and replace broken DNA. The key to optimal health and a long life is keeping DNA healthy, so it produces the cleanest, most accurate cell copies as our cells replicate and reproduce themselves.

The Unified DNA Damage Theory of Aging (UDDTA) asserts that the

basis for controlling and retarding the aging process lies in accurate reproduction of DNA and the ability to keep DNA repair greater than DNA
damage. Without DNA there can be no life, but it endures endless damage
inflicted by environmental toxins, faulty diet, and the physical and mental
stress inherent in modern living. And that damage is directly responsible
for every molecular change that occurs within the body.

The life-threatening diseases most common in Western civilization are
heart disease, stroke, cancer, and dementia, including Alzheimer's disease.
While none of these is exclusively reserved for old age, we become increasingly susceptible to them are we grow older, and all can be ascribed
to the damage to and breakdown of DNA. DNA damage most likely triggers key genetic-control processes such as methylation, altering changes
in our gene profile as we develop from embryo to fetus and then through
childhood, adolescence, adulthood, and into old age.

It is impossible to overstate the importance of healthy DNA. Within
each of the human body's 100 trillion cells is approximately 5 feet of DNA,
which means there are at least a billion miles of DNA in each of us. While
we can be comforted by this fact—for it provides for a huge margin of
error—improving even a small percentage of this vast amount of genetic
material can make a significant difference in the quality of an individual's
health and well-being and in how the person ages. New research has
shown that life spans in both animals and human beings are directly cor-
related with the rate at which DNA can be repaired.

DNA reproduces and replaces itself continually. Under optimal conditions, this reproduction is flawless and every copy is an exact replica of the
one it replaces. This is normally true in children. As we age, however, we are
increasingly vulnerable to factors that damage our DNA during replication.
The body's process of DNA replication is similar to that of a copy machine
making photocopies of an original, with each subsequent copy made from
the previous photocopy. If the copy machine is in perfect condition, the first
copy will hardly be distinguishable from the original. Gradually, though,
even copies made on a good-quality machine will lose definition. A third-
generation copy is slightly less sharp than the original, the fourth-generation
copy even less so, and so forth. Eventually, the process breaks down; it is no
longer possible to make a legible copy, and the message is lost. When this
happens to DNA, the result is the death of a cell.

Thus, the key to optimal health is to keep DNA clean and healthy so that it produces clean and healthy copies of itself. Currently, this can be done by providing the best-possible materials from which to build new DNA, helping the body neutralize excess free radicals and strengthen and nourish cells.

We now know that even in very old people, the telomeres that seem to control the number of times a cell can divide have not reached the terminal positions that signal cell death. This tells us that most people die without having realized their genetic potential. The message of the UDDTA theory, and this book, is that we are programmed for self-repair and longevity. Our understanding of DNA and the way it can be damaged and repaired means that we can choose to live healthy, productive lives beyond our current expectation. We can improve the length of our lives as well as its quality. The power of this information is what *Breaking the Aging Code* is all about.

THREE GOALS FOR FULL GENETIC POTENTIAL

If we are to slow the process by which we age, and live out our full genetic potential, we must adopt these goals:

- To improve the ratio of DNA repair over DNA damage. This will yield fewer cell mutations and more accurate cell copies during cell replication, and will optimize the aging process within all key organs.

- To improve the function of what has been called the aging equation: the processes of glycation, inflammation, oxidation, and methylation, all of which directly affect DNA function, damage, and repair.

- To control and optimize the environmental factors that directly affect DNA. These factors include diet, exercise, and mental state. We can also decrease the negative effects of the environment on aging by reducing toxic elements such as pollution and radiation.

In the next chapter we will look more closely at cell structure and DNA to better understand how microscopic changes on the cellular level can cause major changes—for better or worse—in health and longevity.

CHAPTER 2

Cells, DNA Damage, and DNA Repair

WHEN YOU TEACH YOUR SON,
YOU TEACH YOUR SON'S SON.

—The Talmud

Cells are the basic unit in every organism, from one-celled bacteria to human beings. They make up all of the body's tissues, including skin, organs, bones, nerves, and blood. Cells carry out all of the body's functions. New cells are created by existing cells as the result of cell division, ensuring the continuity of life. Cell division is the mechanism by which traits are passed from one generation to the next. When a cell divides, the genetic material within the so-called parent cell is distributed equally to the two daughter cells, making them genetically identical to the parent. If our cells did not divide and reproduce, we would not grow through the stages of human development. Even when we reach adulthood, cell division remains necessary to replace damaged or dying cells with new, healthy offspring. Depending on their function, some cells divide once a day or even more often. By contrast, some of the most highly specialized cells in the body, such as nerve cells, may not divide at all, although science is beginning to question the long-held assumption that nerve cells that die are never replaced.

The structure and form of a cell depends on its function. Life begins when a sperm cell and an egg cell merge and begin to divide. The growth and development of the embryo and, after eight weeks, the fetus depend on cells dividing and becoming differentiated to form the various tissues of the body. For example, nerve cells send messages throughout the body; some blood cells carry oxygen to all parts of the body; and other blood cells are part of the immune system that works to prevent illness. Cell division, differentiation, and specialization continue until the end of life.

Each cell is like a tiny walled city, full of structures and activity. The wall surrounding it is the *cell membrane*, which allows nutrients to enter and wastes to leave. Inside the membrane wall is a fluid called *cytoplasm* containing water; salts; droplets of fat, and granules of proteins and sugars, all of which provide fuel for the cell's activities; and *nucleic acid*, which holds the patterns for a variety of proteins. There are two varieties of nucleic acids: *deoxyribonucleic acid (DNA)* and *ribonucleic acid (RNA)*. DNA provides the genetic information necessary to form cells, and RNA is instrumental in translating the DNA code into amino acid sequences, which build proteins. The codes themselves are among components within the nucleic acids called *nucleotides.* Also suspended within the cytoplasm are tiny structures called *organelles* (little organs) that play various essential roles in cell function. Among the organelles are *mitochondria*, the cell's power plants, which will be discussed in depth in this chapter. Centrally located in the cell is the *nucleus*, within its own enclosure. The nucleus can be compared to a library containing all the information about our genetic heritage. The information is stored in the form of *chromosomes*, which are made up of the DNA that is the main focus of our quest to promote healthy aging.

CHROMOSOMES, GENES, AND DNA

Continuing the library metaphor, we can think of the human genome as a book containing twenty-three chapters. These are the *chromosomes*. Each chapter contains several thousand stories called *genes*. The stories contain words called *codons*, which are written in letters, known as *bases*, which are part of the nucleotides. There are only four bases: A (adenine), C (cytosine), G (guanine), and T (thymine). Each chromosome is composed of two extremely long molecules of deoxyribonucleic acid (DNA) coiled about each other to form a spiral, or *helix*. Genes are arranged in linear fashion along the DNA strands. The two strands of DNA that make up a chromosome are called a *base pair.* Base pairs are formed by the bonding of A bases with T bases and Gs with Cs. Specific sequences of these paired bases on a DNA strand are called *genes.* Genes provide instructions to our cells about which proteins to synthesize. A gene may be composed of hundreds or even thousands of nucleotides, and a molecule of DNA may contain thousands of genes. The collection of genes is called the *genome.*

The genome can both read and copy itself under the right conditions. The reading process is called *translation* and the copying process is known as *replication.* A single strand of DNA replicates itself by constructing a new strand in which all the Ts are opposite all the As, and all the Gs are opposite all the Cs. When parts of the gene are copied incorrectly or some of the genetic letters are left out, the result is known as a *mutation.*

DNA is also capable of a process called *transcription,* in which the base pair, rather than a single DNA strand, makes an identical copy of itself. The process of transcription makes RNA, in which thymine (T) is replaced by *uracil* (U). RNA is involved in the production of *amino acids,* the building blocks of proteins. The number and sequence of amino acids determine the structure and function of the proteins produced. Certain amino acids are also the precursors of various neurohormones (brain chemicals). Our bodies are primarily composed of proteins. Every protein can be considered a *translated gene.*

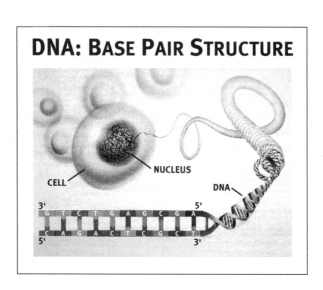

One class of proteins, called *enzymes,* is responsible for all chemical reactions in the body. Enzymes are *catalysts,* which initiate chemical changes in other substances without being changed themselves in the process. We are probably most familiar with the digestive enzymes involved in breaking down foods in the digestive system, and the fermenting enzymes, which are produced by bacteria or yeasts and cause the fermentation of carbohydrates. Fermenting enzymes in the bowel can result in bloating and flatulence; in a properly prepared barrel they create beer.

The cell's nucleus contains twenty-three pairs of chromosomes, one-half of each pair originally derived from the individual's mother's egg cell and the other half from the father's sperm cell. The twenty-third chromosome pair determines a person's sex. If it contains two X chromosomes, the person is female; if it contains one X and one Y chromosome, the person is male.

Genes store coded information for the synthesis of enzymes and hormones as well as proteins. Some proteins regulate the repair of DNA. Others determine which segments of genes are active at a specific time. They turn genes on and off at various stages in the human life cycle and in different parts of the body so cells can perform their assigned functions. Switching genes on and off is referred to as *gene expression* and *suppression.* Specific environmental agents such as radiation, sun exposure, and pollution can modify how genes are expressed or activated. The fundamental goal of anti-aging therapy is to manipulate gene expression to provide healthy maintenance of cell structure and function as we age.

DNA'S JOB DESCRIPTION

Our DNA has plenty of work to do, and, as in any organization, there is a division of labor. Under normal circumstances—that is, in the absence of adverse environmental influences such as toxins, radiation, and pollution—the division of labor is approximately like this:

- 22 percent of our DNA is devoted to synthesizing proteins and RNA.

- 12 percent is devoted to cell division.

- 12 percent controls signaling and communication between cells.

- 12 percent is directly related to immune function.

- 17 percent oversees cell metabolism.

- 8 percent is responsible for maintaining the structural integrity of cells.

- 17 percent has no known function and is known as "junk DNA."

Of course, the scientists who gave the last group that name know it's not junk; they just don't know what it's used for. Several theories exist about junk DNA. One of the earliest is that it is simply extra DNA left over from our evolutionary past. Another is that it provides redundancy, equipping us with extra copies of our genetic code. Redundancy is a familiar concept in human anatomy: it's why we have two kidneys and two lungs. Yet another theory holds that junk DNA may be activated by the earth's and the individual's electromagnetic fields, emotional states, or both. Taking the idea of an emotional component further is the theory that this apparently nonfunctional DNA may respond to focused intentional thought, and may be the basis of the mind-body healing interaction seen in otherwise unexplainable cures or spontaneous remissions. At the moment, all these theories are conjecture, but each is backed by some degree of scientific evidence. We will explore the concept of DNA and mind-body energy interactions in the final chapter of this book.

MITOCHONDRIAL DNA

In addition to the genes found within the nucleus of each cell, other genes exist outside the nucleus, within a cellular organelle called a *mitochondrion*. The mitochondrial genes are inherited only from the mother, which means that human beings have slightly more of their mother's DNA than their father's.

Mitochondria are the cell's power plants. They convert the chemical energy from the food we eat into cellular fuel called *adenosine triphosphate* (ATP) for the body to use. When insulin taps on a cell's door and offers it a delivery of glucose, mitochondria use that glucose to make ATP. Tiny droplets of fat are dealt with in a similar manner. The process by which ATP is formed is essential for all cellular functions, including cell replication. Without ATP, cell repair slows down or stops.

Mitochondria convert the potential chemical energy in food to potential metabolic energy by stripping off the electrons found in the molecules of food and causing them to move through a complex compartment of cellular membranes, as well as through the genes themselves. Mitochondria may be viewed as quantum energy devices that remove energy from matter—the food we eat—and transfer it to different components of the cells, including the nucleus, to create new matter such as proteins and enzymes. The newly created proteins allow cells and organs to grow, reproduce, and maintain health and bodily function. A single ATP molecule must be recycled within a mitochondrion approximately 1,000 times each day for the body to maintain its energy supply.

Nuclear DNA versus Mitochondrial DNA

One of the key features of nuclear DNA is its ability to repair itself as it suffers damage from the environment and from free radicals. Nuclear DNA is different from mitochondrial DNA in that it has a protective layer of proteins called *histones* that absorb much of the free-radical damage and protect the cellular DNA's essential genetic structure and codes. In fact, at the level of the nucleus, a number of DNA repair mechanisms have evolved to prevent severe permanent genetic damage.

Mitochondrial DNA is 2,000 times more susceptible to oxidative damage from free radicals than nuclear DNA. Mitochondrial DNA contains no known repair systems and does not replicate itself. It has no protective histone coat. Mitochondrial DNA is also unique in that it has a ring-shaped structure rather than cellular DNA's double helix. Mitochondrial DNA is also much more susceptible to damage than nuclear DNA because mitochondria are at the site where most free radicals are formed during the process of energy production. Some scientists who study aging consider the functional changes that mitochondria undergo as a consequence of free-radical damage to be a central characteristic of biological aging.

THE IMPORTANCE OF ADULT STEM CELLS

Another kind of cell that deserves mention is the *adult stem cell*. These are not to be confused with *fetal stem cells*, whose use in cloning research is

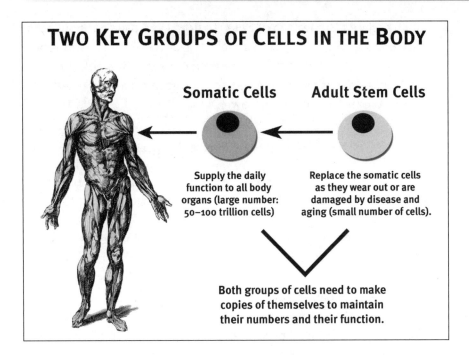

TWO KEY GROUPS OF CELLS IN THE BODY

Somatic Cells

Adult Stem Cells

Supply the daily function to all body organs (large number: 50–100 trillion cells)

Replace the somatic cells as they wear out or are damaged by disease and aging (small number of cells).

Both groups of cells need to make copies of themselves to maintain their numbers and their function.

under considerable controversy. Adult stem cells are found in many different body tissues, including fat, nerve tissue, bone marrow, and the lining of the gut. They carry the genetic code but are not specialized cells that perform a particular function. They can take the form of cells in the tissues where they are needed to restore aging cells and malfunctioning tissues damaged by aging. However, continued damage and poor repair of DNA also injures the genetic coding of adult stem cells, and their regenerative and restorative capacities are eventually lost. Although small in number, the adult stem cells we possess constitute one of the key reservoirs of new cell growth and cell repair as we age. The preservation and restoration of adult stem cell reserves and function will become of paramount importance in the field of anti-aging medicine in the near future.

DNA DAMAGE AND REPAIR: THE FUNDAMENTAL CONCEPT OF THE NEW AGING PARADIGM

While no one can live forever, few people realize their full potential for a long and healthy life. How long we live and how healthy we are in old age are directly related to the ratio of DNA repair to DNA damage in our cells. Heredity plays a role in how effectively our bodies protect and repair DNA, but it is not the whole story. Science has given us the gift of understanding the mechanisms of DNA damage and repair, and the knowledge we need to protect and repair our own DNA.

Mechanism of DNA Repair

Attached to the twenty-three pairs of chromosomes containing our cellular DNA is a substance called the *chromatin layer* that contains the proteins called *histones.* This structure, which resembles a child's Slinky toy, helps stabilize the three-dimensional form of the double helix. More importantly, it protects the genetic content of each chromosome from damage by free radicals and other factors. The chromatin layer is not foolproof, however, and damage does sometimes occur.

Most often damage happens when free radicals penetrate the histones' protective coating, breaking a strand of DNA. This break triggers the release of an enzyme known as *adenosine diphosphate ribosyl transferase,* otherwise known as ADPRT. (You can always recognize an enzyme by the *-ase* suffix.) ADPRT causes the coils of the chromatin layer to spread apart, exposing the chromosome's genes to fluid within the nucleus of the cell. This starts a chain of reparative events: The damaged DNA segments are bathed by several enzymes in the nuclear fluid. Another enzyme *called exonuclease* cuts out the damaged base pairs of the DNA. *DNA polymerase* and *DNA ligase* replace the damaged base pairs with new ones taken from the nuclear cell fluid. *Endonuclease* stitches the DNA thread back together, and the repair is complete. Without the presence of ADPRT, none of this would happen.

Another component of the intracellular fluid is a very important compound known as *nuclear transcription factor kappa B* (NF-κB). NF-κB is activated by oxidative stress. NF-κB inhibits ADPRT from opening the chromatin layer so DNA repair can take place. In this sense NF-κB controls DNA repair by preventing the action of ADPRT. NF-κB also brings about a series of other molecular responses that interfere with DNA repair. If NF-κB can be inhibited, the rate of DNA repair can be markedly improved. NF-κB is also linked to elevated levels of cytokines, immune system cells associated with inflammation. Promising work is underway on a compound that inhibits the action of NF-κB. Among substances shown by recent research to stimulate DNA repair are *zinc* and *niacinamide*, a derivative of the B vitamin niacin. Both of these compounds help ADPRT link to the damaged DNA site so that repair can be completed more quickly and efficiently. A deficiency in the complex of B vitamins or a deficiency in zinc, which can result from an excess of copper in the body, can therefore diminish the body's ability to repair DNA. If the system is low in antioxidants, free radicals have the same negative effect on DNA repair.

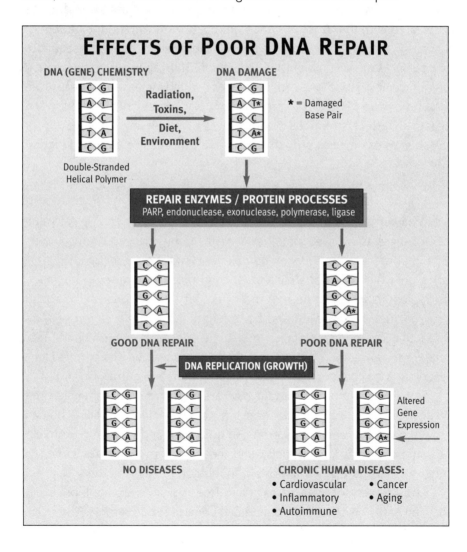

EFFECTS OF POOR DNA REPAIR

Consequences of Poor DNA Repair

DNA damage that is not properly repaired can cause adverse health consequences in several ways. Likely results include inhibition of the methylation process that causes genes to be expressed and inactivated at appropriate times; an increase in glycation; and the creation of free radicals associated with inflammation and chronic disease. Research has disclosed that high levels of DNA damage can make people more susceptible to high blood pressure, elevated levels of blood fats (high cholesterol), atherosclerosis, and coronary artery disease. These are the same diseases associated with the toxic substances in tobacco smoke, and their effect of increasing the population of free radicals. Another potential consequence of poor DNA repair is faulty DNA replication. This can result in the creation of mutagenic disease, or cancer, the risk of which increases with age. Even if mutations don't occur, the presence of poor copies of cells directly and negatively affects stem-cell-pool reserves by increasing deterioration of the sources of new cell growth responsible for repair to damaged organs.

DNA Damage: A Biomarker of Aging

A biomarker is a measurable chemical substance or physiological value that changes as we age. Some biomarkers can be changed through intervention; others cannot. *Nonmodifiable biomarkers* are genetic characteristics on which diet, pharmaceuticals, nutraceuticals (medicines made from plants), and lifestyle have no effect, at least at present. In adults these include body height and bone length. *Modifiable biomarkers* are those that respond to changes in lifestyle, diet, and environmental factors. For instance, muscle mass and aerobic capacity can be improved fairly rapidly with changes in exercise patterns, diet, and nutrition.

Some of the more important biomarkers that have an effect on the quality of life are the endocrine hormones, including DHEA, human growth hormone, and testosterone, in both men and women. Skin thickness and elasticity, lung capacity, and the ratio of muscle mass to fat are other biomarkers that are important in relation to aging.

Measurement of DNA damage and free-radical levels are biomarkers that can easily be obtained from a small urine or blood sample. They supply key information to document the effectiveness of an age-management program.

The Importance of Improving DNA Repair Processes

The reason people do not realize their full health and longevity potential is not faulty DNA but imperfect DNA repair processes. This results in poor genetic copies in each generation of cell replication and causes mutations in proteins and errors in enzyme production. It is essential to keep in mind the effects of today's progressively hostile environment, including oxidative stress, huge numbers of free radicals, and consequent damage to both nuclear and mitochondrial DNA. There are many things you can do to improve your body's ability to repair damaged DNA, as this book explains.

CHAPTER 3

Biomarkers of Aging

SOMETIMES THE OBVIOUS CAN STARE YOU IN THE FACE.

—*Matt Ridley, Genome*

There's probably not an adult alive who hasn't had the experience of seeing an acquaintance for the first time in years and being shocked by how old that person looks. The shock reminds us that we, too, are aging. We don't see the signs as clearly in ourselves, even though we see our own faces and bodies in the mirror every day, because the changes occur so gradually. It's only when we encounter someone we haven't seen in a long time that the recognition of our own inevitable mortality strikes with unpleasant force.

While we notice wrinkles, bifocals, and other visible manifestations of aging, we tend to overlook the many internal factors that control the rate at which we age. Just as we can measure more readily seen characteristics, we can also monitor our own aging by assessing our *biological terrain,* the totality of our internal biochemical environment. Taken together, these factors are the *biomarkers of aging.* A biomarker is a measurable chemical substance or physiological value that is known to change over time. By improving our biomarkers we improve our health in general and our DNA repair and longevity in particular.

Some biomarkers are objective—that is, they are measurable and not subject to opinion. Others are subjective—they depend on perceptions rather than verifiable facts. Some biomarkers can be modified while others cannot be changed. This chapter discusses a variety of biomarkers and describes the significance of the information they provide. Later in the book you will learn techniques to modify and improve many of your biomarkers.

OBJECTIVE AND SUBJECTIVE BIOMARKERS

Objective biomarkers provide hard data, measured and documented with standardized and accepted laboratory technology. They can be considered direct measurements of gene expression. Changes in the functions of genes and the proteins they produce are responsible for creating the molecular changes that we see in objective biomarker measurements.

Some of the more important objective biomarkers that determine quality of life, as well as appearance, are the secretions of the *endocrine glands.* These glands synthesize hormones and deliver them directly into the blood or lymph, through which they are circulated to all parts of the body. The endocrine glands include the pituitary, thyroid, parathyroids, adrenals, pancreas, and the sex glands—the ovaries and testes. The lining of the gastrointestinal tract also performs endocrine functions. The hypothalamus produces hormones that affect the production of some of the endocrine hormones. These hormones will be discussed later in this chapter and explored in greater detail in Chapter 5.

Each hormone has a specific effect on some part of the body, or a general effect on the body as a whole. Its presence in our systems in sufficient quantities and its relative balance to the other hormones is crucial to the quality of our lives. Too much or too little of a specific hormone is apt to trigger an excess or deficiency of some or all of the rest. Hormones both affect and are affected by gene expression. A hormone panel, performed in a laboratory on a blood sample, is the way the relative balance of the endocrine hormones is measured. Any physician can draw the blood and order the tests, but the analysis of results as they affect aging is usually best done by someone skilled in the techniques of aging management.

Among other objective biomarkers are measurements of the pH level (relative acidity or alkalinity) of the blood, cardiovascular fitness, and body weight in relation to height (the body mass index, or BMI). A bone density scan to look for the presence of osteoporosis is an important measurement for both women and men. It is a myth that only women are prone to develop osteoporosis. Men are less subject to it because their bones are more dense to begin with, but after age seventy-five the risk to men is as great as it is to women. The results of tests for glycation, inflammation, oxidation, and methylation are among the most important biomarkers we can obtain in relation to DNA damage and gene expression.

Subjective biomarkers are generally a reflection of indirect secondary gene expression changes; that is, they are measures of the symptoms and effects a patient may sense or feel, which are related indirectly to the molecular and genetic changes that cause them. Subjective biomarkers are largely drawn from the individual's perceptions of age-related change, for better or for worse. They can be tracked in a journal, or revealed by answering questions about signs and symptoms related to aging. (Signs can be observed by anyone; symptoms are not visible to others and must be reported by the individual.) Physicians who specialize in aging management often use questionnaires to get their patients' perceptions. The questionnaires may include one on family health history, to screen for inherited genetic tendencies likely to manifest themselves in response to specific lifestyle choices. The family history questionnaire is often paired with one relating to lifestyle, behavioral tendencies, and the social and physical environment in which the individual lives.

By recording the combination of objective laboratory data and subjective observation of changes, we can monitor the utility and effectiveness of an anti-aging program with a high degree of scientific credibility. Photographic documentation is an extremely important tool in a comprehensive age-management evaluation. It is an unblinking physical representation of the individual and reflects the combined effect of the underlying changes in genetic expression that have taken place during one's lifetime.

MODIFIABLE AND NONMODIFIABLE BIOMARKERS

Another convenient way of looking at the biomarkers of aging is to determine which can be modified and which cannot. Nonmodifiable biomarkers are genetic characteristics that no amount of anti-aging intervention will change, such as body height, bone length, and whether one has five or six lumbar (low back) vertebra.

Modifiable biomarkers are those that respond relatively quickly to changes in lifestyle, diet, and other environmental factors. For instance, decreased muscle mass and diminished aerobic capacity are strongly cor-related to a higher biological age. But they are also two of the biomarkers that can be improved quickly with changes in exercise regimen and with appropriate modifications in diet and nutrition. Muscular strength, basal metabolic rate, the ratio of muscle to fat, glucose tolerance, blood fats (cholesterol, triglycerides, and low- and high-density lipoprotein, also called LDL and HDL, levels), blood pressure, and bone density are also modifiable biomarkers that respond to lifestyle interventions, including changes in diet, nutrient supplements, and prescription medications.

Laboratory tests exist that monitor free-radical levels and DNA dam-age, both of which are easily sampled in blood or urine. Attention to these test results has been positively correlated to marked improvements in health and well-being. Among other measurable and modifiable bio-markers are changes in the four factors that make up the aging equation: rates of glycation, methylation, oxidative stress, and inflammation. Improve-ments in the results of these laboratory tests are directly related to over-all improvements in gene expression at the cellular level.

SNPs

The DNA of any two individuals is about 99.9 percent identical, yet each of us, except for identical twins, is genetically unique. The crucial differ-ence is in that last one-tenth of 1 percent of our genes, which are termed *single nucleotide polymorphisms,* or SNPs (pronounced "snips"). Although they are not modifiable, SNPs may be the mother of all biomarkers. If you think of DNA as a string of the letters A, G, C, and T (3 billion of them) and compare the DNA of any two people, you will occasionally find places where a letter differs between the two strings. These variations are SNPs. They occur, on average, once in every 2,000 letters in a string of DNA.

Scientists have only just begun to explore the implications of SNPs. Not only do SNPs account for variations in our physical appearance, but they also seem to explain why people react differently to the same medication. Since SNPs can affect the nature of proteins and enzymes that genes synthesize, it makes sense to assume that these minute genetic variations can influence how we absorb and metabolize medications. And if the way we react to medicine is influenced in this way, it makes sense to assume that we will have varying reactions to the food we eat and to the nutritional supplements we take.

Obtaining a DNA sample for testing is a simple matter of swabbing or lightly scraping the inside of the cheek. Actually, your toothbrush is a rich source of DNA, as anyone who watches any of the immensely popular television shows based on forensic investigation knows. SNP testing is already being done; observers predict that it will be commonplace by 2010. The resulting information will be invaluable in designing highly customized nutrient-based therapies. For example, a person whose SNPs show a propensity for developing prostate cancer might be advised early in life to take extra zinc or saw palmetto supplements. Someone prone to loss of calcium in the bones could be given calcium supplementation to prevent osteoporosis. Tendencies toward poor cardiac and circulatory health could be minimized, immune system deficiencies overcome, and susceptibility to oxidative stress neutralized. SNPs can also indicate when nutritional supplements are unnecessary. The possibilities for using such data are virtually endless.

Modifiable Biomarkers

The rest of the biomarkers discussed here are less dramatic in scope, but all can be modified in relatively easy and productive ways.

Acidity/Alkalinity

A key component of our internal biochemical environment is the degree of acidity or alkalinity of our blood. In chemistry, the acidity or alkalinity of a substance is expressed as a pH (potential of hydrogen) value. The pH value is a measurement of the activity and potential energy found within the hydrogen ion. As hydrogen concentration increases, pH decreases and the substance becomes more acidic. A pH of 7.0 is neutral, indicating that it is neither acidic nor alkaline. A number smaller than 7.0 indicates relative acidity, a number larger than 7.0 means the substance is alkaline. Maximum acidity has a pH value of 0, maximum alkalinity ranks at 14. The pH scale is logarithmic, so the difference between each unit on the scale is tenfold. A pH of 5.0 is ten times more acidic than a pH of 6.0 and a pH of 4.0 is one hundred times more acidic.

The body's various tissues and fluids operate best at different pH levels, each more or less finely circumscribed if proper biochemical function is to be preserved. For example, the pH of saliva is between 6.0 and 7.0, neutral to slightly acidic. Stomach juices have a pH ranging from 1.0 to 3.5 and are thus very acidic. The secretions of the small intestine tend toward the alkaline at 7.5 to 8.0. The pH of blood has the smallest range, with arterial blood having a pH of 7.4 to 7.45, and venous blood a pH of 7.3 to 7.35. The difference in the values for blood is related to the higher concentration of oxygen in arterial blood.

Because our cells require a pH within a very narrow range, if the pH of any fluid or tissue falls outside the prescribed range, cellular function is compromised. When pH decreases to a point outside of range, a condition known as acidosis is created; a higher-than-normal pH results in alkalosis. At the extreme, an out-of-range pH value will result in death. Our bodies have an intricate array of mechanisms to maintain proper pH values, but environmental toxins and even improper dietary intake can compromise these mechanisms. For example, excessive consumption of acidic foods can start a chain of events that can be felt in the digestive system, in the immune system, and even in the lymphatic system. But many lesser imbalances do their damage in silence. Therefore, measuring the pH of blood and saliva can yield biomarkers that provide important information and suggest remedial measures.

Body Mass Index

Because being overweight can increase the risk of developing such conditions as cardiovascular disease, osteoarthritis, and diabetes, it's important to maintain a healthy body weight at all stages of life. Body mass index (BMI) measures body weight in relation to height and is a means of monitoring your progress as you work on losing (or gaining) weight. The idea is simple: as your weight increases, so does your BMI. You can use the formula on page 40 to determine your BMI.

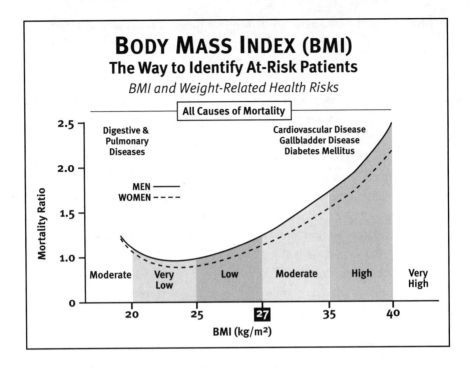

BODY MASS INDEX (BMI)
The Way to Identify At-Risk Patients
BMI and Weight-Related Health Risks

Sample BMI Calculation

(1) Weight nude (in pounds) = 194

(2) Divide (1) by 2.2 to get equivalent in kilograms = 88.2

(3) Barefoot height 69 inches

(4) Divide (3) by 39.4 to get equivalent in meters = 1.75

(5) Multiply (4) by itself = 3.1

(6) Divide (2) by (5) to get BMI = 28.5

Interpreting the results:

Women	Men	Verdict
<20	<21	Underweight
21–23	22–24	Optimal
24–26	25–27	Cautionary
27–31	28–32	Overweight
>31	>32	Obese

BMI = weight (in kilograms) divided by height (in meters, squared)
(Divide your height in centimeters by 100 to get height in meters,
then square that number.)

Generally, a BMI between 21 and 24 for women and between 22 and 25 for men improves your chances for a long and healthy life. However, if your body is more muscular than most, your BMI will tend toward the higher end of the range or even fall above the recommended standard, because muscle is heavier than fat. Therefore, BMI is not the most accurate way of assessing the percentage of body fat compared to lean muscle. The relationship between BMI and percent of muscle mass varies, depending on gender and age. Women tend to have a higher percentage of body fat than men with the same BMI, and older people may have a higher percentage of body fat than younger people with the same BMI.

Therefore, in addition to using the BMI measurement to determine your ideal weight, you may also want to measure your muscle to fat ratio. This can be done by a healthcare professional or health-club instructor using a pair of calipers, an instrument for measuring thickness. As a quick measurement, you can pinch the flesh at your waist on one side. The rule of thumb is that if you pinch an inch or more, you're carrying more body fat than is good for you.

Muscle Strength

With advancing age comes a corresponding decline in muscle mass, and as a result, muscle strength. In fact, it's estimated that by age sixty-five, many people have lost up to 30 percent of their muscle mass. Because muscle cells don't divide, muscle mass depends on the size of the individual muscle cells, rather than their number.

It's believed that the age-related decline of such hormones as human growth hormone (HGH), insulinlike growth factor (IGF-1), and testosterone is responsible for some of the loss of muscle mass that occurs with advancing age. When stimulated, these hormones are responsible for improving muscle strength by helping to repair damaged muscle tissue, and for increasing muscle mass while decreasing body fat. As levels of hormones decrease with age, however, the processes of muscle-cell repair and growth become less effective. Although you can buy HGH in some stores and on the Internet, this is not a hormone that you can experiment with safely. If you think you can benefit from increased growth hormone, be sure to work with a health professional.

Diabetes, Glucose Tolerance, and Insulin Resistance

With age, the body becomes less effective in taking up glucose (sugar) from the bloodstream to use as energy for body cells. Glucose that cannot be stored in the cells is stored as body fat or blood fats (serum cholesterol). In response to chronically elevated blood sugar levels, the pancreas releases more and more insulin to bring glucose levels back under control. Cells become so resistant to insulin over time that they can no longer effectively accept glucose from the blood, a condition known as insulin resistance or glucose intolerance. This condition can develop into Type 2 diabetes if it is left untreated. Insulin resistance is also associated with high blood pressure, atherosclerosis, heart attack, and stroke.

Blood sugar levels are easy to assess. One simple test, available at any drugstore, consists of a strip that is dipped into a urine specimen. The resulting color of the strip gives a rough indication of whether or not there is too much glucose in your blood. If there is, it will spill over into your urine. You need to see a physician as soon as possible if that seems to be the case, because you may have diabetes. Even if the urine test appears normal, it's a good idea to have a professional screening for high blood sugar once a year. Diabetes can exist without symptoms for years before it becomes evident. The effects of elevated blood sugar can still be doing damage to nerves and blood vessels during those years, causing a painful condition called neuropathy.

A glucose tolerance test shows how efficient your body is at handling sugar. It is done in a laboratory after twelve hours without food. A standard amount of glucose is given as a drink or injected into a vein. Blood samples are then drawn hourly and analyzed to determine your ability to metabolize sugar. The test may last for two to six hours; the longer period is used when insulin resistance is suspected.

Another way to test for insulin resistance is to check the urine for C-peptide, a byproduct of insulin that indicates how much insulin the pancreas is producing. People who produce no insulin have no C-peptide. Those who produce too much because they are insulin resistant have elevated C-peptide levels. Since insulin resistance commonly leads to Type 2 diabetes, and most people's resistance to insulin increases with age, watching out for insulin resistance is an important part of any anti-aging program. If you discover you are insulin resistant, or even a Type 2 diabetic, you'll be happy to know there is much you can do to mitigate the results.

Cholesterol

We hear a lot about the importance of reducing cholesterol levels in maintaining good health, but cholesterol is not always harmful. In fact, it is essential to the proper function of the body because it plays a role in building cell membranes and producing hormones, among other things. Problems arise when levels of cholesterol in the body exceed the amount needed for body functions, but problems also arise when the serum cholesterol level is too low.

Most of the body's cholesterol is produced by the liver and travels through the bloodstream in particles called lipoproteins to its targets throughout the body. There are two kinds of lipoproteins: low-density lipoproteins (LDL), which transport cholesterol to the cells of the body, and high-density lipoprotein (HDL), which remove excess cholesterol from the blood and tissues. LDL cholesterol is known as the "bad" cholesterol because it can build up on artery walls, forming plaques that can block arteries and cause heart attacks and strokes. This type of cholesterol is also highly susceptible to oxidative stress. On the other hand, HDL is known as the "good" cholesterol because of its role in reducing an excess level of LDL cholesterol. Good health, therefore, depends not so much on reducing cholesterol levels as a whole, but on balancing LDL and HDL cholesterol.

Blood Pressure

Blood pressure measures the force exerted by the blood on the walls of your blood vessels. Two numbers are used to express blood pressure, and the two are combined to make a fraction. The top number shows systolic blood pressure, which is measured at the point when the heart muscle is contracting, or beating. Diastolic blood pressure, the bottom number of the fraction, is measured when the heart relaxes between beats. In general, 120/80 is considered to be a normal blood pressure reading. A systolic measure of 140 or more, or a diastolic measure over 99 is indicative of high blood pressure.

High blood pressure, or hypertension, causes the heart to work harder to pump blood through the circulatory system and increases the risk of kidney failure, heart attack, and stroke. Conditions such as obesity, insulin resistance, diabetes, and an overactive thyroid gland increase the risk of developing high blood pressure. Additionally, unhealthy habits such as tobacco use, consumption of caffeine and other stimulants, and a high intake of sodium may also increase the risk of hypertension.

Bone Density

Bone is living tissue composed of calcium and other essential minerals, plus protein. There are two types of bone cells: osteoclasts are responsible for breaking down old bone, and osteoblasts make new bone. The entire process by which bone is broken down and then rebuilt is called remodeling, and it continues throughout life.

In our younger years, the remodeling process ensures that bone is made faster than it is broken down, keeping our bones strong, or dense, and healthy. However, beginning in our late thirties or early forties, the balance of bone loss and bone growth shifts, and remodeling does not replace bone at the same rate that it is broken down. This results in a steady decline in total bone mass. Bones become weakened and brittle over time, leading to a greater risk of fractures and breaks. Osteoporosis, or brittle bone disease, is the result of decreased bone density.

THE IMPORTANCE OF BIOMARKERS

Measuring biomarkers of aging allows us to monitor the impact of DNA damage and repair, because observable changes to biomarkers are manifestations of changes in gene expression. The goal of an age-management program is to improve modifiable biomarkers, by making dietary and lifestyle changes and implementing an appropriate nutritional supplementation program. Rather than merely addressing the visible signs of aging, we can now begin to work on the source of aging: changes in DNA and gene expression. We are able to track the progression of the aging process because it's possible to measure many of the biomarkers of aging. In cases where biomarkers are modifiable some simple lifestyle changes can have a profound impact on quality of life and longevity. The later chapters in this book are devoted to the measures you can take to combat aging and extend your life.

BODY CHANGES THAT ACCOMPANY AGING

The physical changes we observe as we age are due to the aging equation described throughout this book. These changes are due to alterations in gene-expression patterns over time. The noticeable physical changes in different areas of the body can be halted, and in some cases reversed, with both anti-aging nutritional and medical therapy and with cosmetic surgical procedures, where necessary, bringing about a combination of improved health and improved appearance. A convenient way to understand the fundamental relationships of the aging process is to examine its effect on each area of the body.

The Face

Typically, the most visible change associated with aging is seen in the face, where the loss of elasticity of the skin results in wrinkles and creases. Altered gene expression results in a changed ratio of collagen and elastin, the substances that give the skin its firmness and pliability. An important biochemical cause of this change is the constant elevation of blood glucose levels, resulting in glycation and cross-linking of skin proteins. This is how wrinkles are born. Faulty nutrition makes blood sugar levels unstable, paticularly when the tendency is to eat on the run and emphasize easy-to-grab foods high in carbohydrates. When glucose rises and then drops rapidly, as it does in insulin resistance, the body releases cortisol, a stress hormone, to bring the blood sugar level back up. This hormonal roller coaster causes cell damage and often results in facial skin tone that outpaces a person's chronological age. Elevated cortisol levels also cause the loss of the fat layer underlying the skin, resulting in other facial changes.

The wrinkled neck so characteristic of advancing age is caused by a decrease in muscle tone and collagen in the neck, as well as lessening elasticity of the skin. DNA damage due to elevated levels of free radicals results in a decrease in the synthesis of collagen. Another component of collagen loss is cell inflammation that is not detectable by testing. Decreases in key hormones that occur as part of the normal aging process also affect tissues of the face and neck, including declining secretions of testosterone, estrogen, progesterone, growth hormone, and thyroid hormones.

The Torso

Within the torso, or truncal region, aging changes include loss of muscle tone and the abnormal appearance of excess body fat. Lipodystrophy, defective fat metabolism, is one of the results of insulin resistance. Its effect is seen most often in the abdomen, and potbellies become increasingly common as we age. To make matters worse, a decline in muscle mass occurs with aging as growth-hormone and testosterone levels, in women as well as in men, decline.

In women, not only do levels of estrogen and progesterone decline after menopause, but also the balance between them shifts in a way that causes a buildup of fat, especially on the abdomen, hips, and thighs. Abdominal fat is stored in an organ called the omentum, which looks like lace interspersed with lumps of chicken fat.

The Male Chest

In men, gynecomastia—the development of enlarged mammary glands— becomes increasingly common with age as the result of excess body fat in the upper chest and breast area. Gynecomastia is also associated with the decrease in muscle-maintaining hormones, particularly testosterone and growth hormone. Excess fat in the breast area is apt to be both a cause and a result of gynecomastia because fat cells synthesize estrogen in men as well as in women.

The Female Chest

In women, two types of breast-related changes can occur. The first, breast enlargement, is frequently associated with abnormal levels of either progesterone or estrogen since inappropriate ratios produce continued growth of breast tissue. This can occur early in adolescence or later in life. At the other extreme, the loss of appropriate progesterone and estrogen levels result in drooping breasts or a significant reduction in breast size. Changes in breast structure are related to changes in the milk glands and associated tissues when the childbearing years are over. As throughout the body, there is also a loss of collagen and degradation of elastin, the connective tissue fibers that give skin its elasticity. Both are associated with decreased insulin sensitivity.

ESTABLISHING A BASELINE ON AGING

The biomarkers of aging give us a way to establish a baseline when we begin our anti-aging program, and to track our progress over time. Putting our focus on the modifiable biomarkers gives us a way to set goals, as well as to monitor results. We can also reverse some of the visible changes associated with aging and increase the firmness and elasticity of skin and muscles by improving the ratio of DNA repair to DNA damage. Insulin resistance can also be reversed, enhancing both biomarkers and appearance. The next chapter explains how an anti-aging program manages the aging equation by controlling glycation, inflammation, oxidation, and methylation.

CHAPTER 4

The Aging Equation: Glycation, Inflammation, Oxidation, and Methylation

IF I KNEW I WOULD LIVE AS LONG AS I HAVE,
I WOULD HAVE TAKEN BETTER CARE OF MYSELF.
—*Comedian George Burns, at age 101*

The four processes that make up the aging equation—glycation, inflammation, oxidation, and methylation—are natural processes. To some extent, they are all unavoidable. What makes us focus on them is the fact that most of us make lifestyle choices that exaggerate their effects and cause us to age prematurely. An understanding of how these processes work at the cellular level and their effects on DNA damage and repair is important, if we are to learn how to control them and live as long as we can in the best possible health.

GLYCATION

Glycation, also known as *non-enzymatic glycolysation,* is a destructive process that continually occurs throughout our bodies. It cannot be avoided, but it can and must be minimized as part of the anti-aging regimen. Glycation occurs when a glucose molecule binds to a protein molecule. The result is a damaged protein unable to perform any useful function. Mechanisms exist to keep glycation under control in a healthy person with normal, well-regulated blood sugars, but as we age it becomes increasingly difficult to keep blood sugar levels under control. If we are not careful, glycation can become a major cause of aging and of health problems that can include diabetes and cancer. The cross-linking of proteins with glucose molecules that is characteristic of glycation is associated with insulin resistance, the failure of insulin to do its primary job.

Carbohydrates and a small fraction of the protein we eat turns into glucose when digested. When glucose enters the bloodstream, the pancreas sends insulin to round up the glucose molecules and tuck them into the body's cells to be turned into energy, as needed. This storage is accomplished through places on the cell walls known as *receptors*. The receptors are the same size and shape as a glucose molecule; molecules and receptors fit together much the way jigsaw puzzle pieces do. When a glucose molecule is deformed by glycation, it no longer fits a receptor. Cells are deprived of energy and glucose remains in the bloodstream longer than it should. It is eventually stored as fat, either in tissues or in the blood as serum cholesterol. When cells are unable to accept insulin's offer of glucose, the pancreas responds by secreting even more insulin. The result is called insulin resistance, and it is characterized by excessive levels of insulin in the blood. Glycation is the process that brings about this chronic condition and its serious implications for health and aging.

Insulin is but one of the hormones affected by glycation. Hormones, the chemicals that carry signals to activate and control our organs, are also proteins. Glucose molecules attach themselves to hormones and deform them, making the necessary snug fit with their receptors impossible. In this way, the signals of anti-aging hormones such as the adrenal hormone dehydroepiandrosterone (DHEA), human growth hormone, and insulinlike growth factor (IGF-1), are diminished, and their messages do not get through to the cells that need their instructions.

These effects and others result from the excessive presence of glucose in the bloodstream. Excessive blood glucose is a consequence of the typical American diet, which is high in sugars and starches. Receptor sites on the cell surface become steadily less sensitive to insulin as we age. When coupled with a diet that produces more glucose than we need, the result is inevitable: glycation, insulin resistance, and, as the pancreas is forced to overwork to get cells to respond to insulin's signals, the likelihood of diabetes. In this way, high glucose levels interfere with the fundamental processes of life.

AGEs and Aging

The cross-linked molecules that glycation produces are known as *advanced glycation end-products*, or AGEs. It's the AGEs that age us. No other molecule is as toxic to proteins as AGEs. Cross-linkage toughens tissues and deprives them of their elasticity. Nowhere is this more visible than in the damage AGEs do to collagen. Collagen is the most abundant protein in the human body, representing about 30 percent of total body protein. Its fibers are found in the connective tissue of bone, ligaments, cartilage, and skin. Collagen is abundant even in our teeth (except for the enamel) and forms the ligaments that hold our teeth in their sockets. Glycation disrupts the function of organs that are meant to be flexible. It hardens arteries. It stiffens myosin, the protein in muscle fibers, affecting the structure and function of muscles and impairing strength and flexibility. AGEs inflict damage on the tiny filters in the kidneys, causing the renal disease so often associated with diabetes. Glycation and its end-products are responsible for damage to the retina. Stiffening of the lens of the eye and the formation of cataracts can be traced to glycation. Neuropathy, whether by itself or associated with diabetes, is associated with glycation.

When glycation strikes immunoglobulin (Ig), an immune system antibody in the blood, the Ig molecule's shape is changed and its function is impaired. Two results are possible: autoimmune reactions such as rheumatoid arthritis and lupus, and an increased vulnerability to infection.

Look at the list of harmful effects of glycation: damage to the eyes, kidneys, peripheral nerves, and blood vessels; malfunction of the immune system; failure of insulin to store glucose as energy with resulting muscle fatigue, high cholesterol, and the added risk of heart attack and stroke. All these consequences of glycation are also associated with Type 2 (insulin-resistant) diabetes. All are also associated with aging, which explains why diabetics tend to age prematurely. But you don't have to be diabetic to suffer the ill effects of glycation. All it takes is overconsumption of starches and sugars, leading to an overabundance of glucose in the blood.

But that's not all: AGEs are virtual free-radical factories. And chronically elevated serum insulin is an important cause of inflammation, the second of the four factors in the aging equation. To complete the picture, cross-linked proteins inhibit effective DNA repair. Glycation, therefore, is at the heart of the aging equation.

INFLAMMATION

No one is a stranger to acute inflammation—the redness, heat, swelling, and pain associated with injury. It makes no difference whether the injury is caused by physical trauma, a pathogenic organism (a germ or bacterium), a foreign body, blockage in a blood vessel, exposure to radiation, or extremely high or low temperature (burning or freezing). The word "acute" means sharp and severe; acute inflammation comes on suddenly and is of limited duration. Acute inflammation is a normal part of the body's immune response and is part of the healing process. It begins with dilation of the blood vessels at the site of the injury, leading to an increase in blood flow, the cause of the redness and heat. The capillaries become more permeable, allowing blood plasma to move into the injured tissues but also causing swelling and pain, the result of pressure on nerve endings. Immune system cells and other healing chemicals in the plasma infuse the area, and healing begins. Typically the worst of the redness, heat, swelling, and pain starts to diminish within twelve hours.

When we think of chronic inflammation, we tend to think of auto-immune diseases such as rheumatoid arthritis in which there are also episodes of acute inflammation, and the pain is more or less constant. The autoimmune response occurs when immune cells mistakenly identify tis-sue molecules as outside invaders and create antibodies to attack them. Once the immune system has identified something as foreign, whether correctly or not, it doesn't forget, and from then on the antibodies are always ready for a fight. Chronic inflammation is generally assumed to be accompanied intermittently by redness, heat, swelling, and pain. The inflammatory response may come and go, but it never fully disappears. Nonsteroidal anti-inflammatory drugs (NSAIDs) such as aspirin, ibuprofen, and naproxyn often alleviate the symptoms. When NSAIDs fail, physicians may recommend a more radical alternative: corticosteroids to weaken or immobilize the immune system.

There is another kind of chronic inflammation related to our interest in aging management. The term for it is *chronic subclinical inflammation.*

It is the underlying cause of a long list of familiar diseases that are not commonly associated in the public mind with inflammation. Diabetes of both types can cause and be caused by chronic subclinical inflammation. The same is true of atherosclerosis (hardening of the arteries), heart valve dysfunction, obesity, congestive heart failure, and digestive system diseases such as Crohn's disease. Diseases that involve subclinical inflammation usually follow a circular path, acting as both cause and effect. They feed on themselves in a downward spiral unless some healing influence intervenes. As in all forms of chronic inflammation, immune system cells are involved, but they may present no signs or symptoms until serious damage has been done.

As we age, hidden inflammation poses an increasing threat to health, and to life itself. Aging diminishes our built-in defense system against chronic inflammation. Faulty diet and poor lifestyle choices make matters even worse. Understanding the mechanisms of chronic subclinical inflammation may enable you to make better lifestyle choices in the future.

One of the most potent forces related to subclinical inflammation is chronic elevated blood sugar, whether or not it has risen to the level of diabetes. High blood sugar triggers elevated levels of insulin in the blood, and hyperinsulinemia is proinflammatory.

The glycation of proteins is one of the greatest forces driving chronic inflammation. Every doughnut, candy bar, and soda adds to the toxic excess of dietary glucose. Bathing cells in sugar produces an inflammatory state. AGEs attack collagen (connective tissue) cells. Many inflammatory diseases, lupus among them, involve damage to connective tissue. Lest this sound like a diatribe against sugar-containing foods alone, you should know that frying and other techniques that cook foods at high temperatures also contribute to glycation, promoting inflammation.

Eicosanoids and Cytokines

Two kinds of immune system cells are associated with inflammation: *eicosanoids* and *cytokines*. Eicosanoids come in three varieties: prostaglandins, leukotrienes, and thromboxanes. Like hormones, eicosanoids are chemical messengers that influence various body functions. Unlike hormones, which are secreted by glands and move through the bloodstream to deliver their messages, eicosanoids are produced and do their work within the cells. What they do depends on the type of cell that produced them. Eicosanoids have a very short life span and are destroyed by enzymes too quickly to be measured by a laboratory test. But just because they don't stay around for long doesn't mean they don't have a profound effect on your health and the rate at which you age.

Eicosanoids can be considered "good" or "bad," depending on how they behave. They are involved in many body functions, including blood pressure, the breaking down of fats, fluid balance and swelling, clotting, sexual potency in men, uterine contractions in menstruation and child-birth, the secretion of stomach acids, the dilation of blood vessels and air chambers in the lungs, the signaling of pain, fever, the operation of the immune system, and—most importantly to people interested in anti-aging—inflammation. Good eicosanoids control the proliferation of cells, working to prevent cancer. Bad eicosanoids take some of the blame for osteoporosis. Even bad eicosanoids can be good, if they are not present in excessive quantities. For example, the bad eicosanoids are involved in deep vein thrombosis (DVT), the formation of blood clots in veins, a life-threatening disease. But these same eicosanoids control clotting, and pro-tect us from bleeding to death.

Eicosanoids are synthesized from the breakdown of arachidonic acid, a fatty acid that comes from the fat in red meat, organ meats, and egg yolks. A diet high in sugars and starches also encourages the production of arachidonic acid. You need some arachidonic acid, but an overload encourages production of inflammatory eicosanoids. Other essential fatty acids (EFAs) come into play in building both good and bad eicos-anoids. EFAs come from dietary fat, and because they are important to the health of your cells, you want a liberal supply of them. Whether your eicosanoids are predominantly good or bad depends in large part on the ratio in your bloodstream of insulin and glucagon, the hormone that decreases when insulin increases. Insulin plays an important role in stimu-lating the development of bad eicosanoids while glucagon promotes the production of good eicosanoids. Inflammation results when eicosanoids are out of balance.

Inflammation also results when you have an excess of immune system cells known as *inflammatory cytokines.* These destructive cell-signaling chemicals promote inflammation and contribute to the development of many degenerative autoimmune diseases, as well as to cardiovascular disease, cancer, and diabetes. Arachidonic acid plays a role in the creation of cytokines as well as eicosanoids. But injury and infection also trigger cytokine release as the body works to heal itself. The involvement of cytokines in inflammation is simply a matter of too much of a good thing.

If you've ever noticed that you feel achy and sore when you haven't had enough sleep, here's why: Lack of restful, restorative sleep results in an excess of cytokines, and cytokines cause muscles to ache. Most Americans are chronically sleep deprived, setting themselves up for chronic inflammation and premature aging. The major symptoms of fibromyalgia, a chronic condition characterized by nonrestorative sleep and musculoskeletal pain, are a common result of excessive cytokine production in those who are genetically predisposed to the condition. The muscle aches often associated with diabetes are another example of cytokine overload. Excess insulin is associated with overproduction of cytokines, and excess cytokines cause inflammation.

Cytokine overload has another effect that is often characteristic of aging: cognitive dysfunction, a decrease in short-term memory and the ability to think things through. The brain chemical most closely associated with memory and thinking is acetylcholine. Cytokines inhibit the action of acetylcholine and can bring about episodes of "brain fog." Acetylcholine is also responsible for carrying messages between the voluntary nerves and muscles. When cytokines interfere with the action of acetylcholine, poor coordination and muscular weakness result. All of these problems can be caused by the chronic inflammatory process that comes from a high-sugar diet and its resulting excess of insulin.

OXIDATION

Oxygen in our cells combines with glucose and fat to produce energy. The process takes place in the mitochondria, the tiny power plants within our cells that produce the chemical adenosine triphosphate (ATP). ATP powers a wide variety of cellular activities. Oxygen is required when energy is produced, whether it is in our cells, the engine of an automobile, or the furnace that heats your home. To put out a fire, you smother it to deprive it of oxygen. Oxygen molecules give up electrons and become unstable when burning, or energy release, occurs. This process is known as oxidation. It is a natural process necessary to the continuation of life. Oxidation also takes place in inorganic materials. Rust on metal is the result of oxidation. Since rust ruins metal, oxidation is obviously a mixed blessing. Just as we can see the oxidative damage on metal, we can see it in ourselves in the facial wrinkles we develop as we grow older. Oxidative damage takes place within our cells, too. It is the primary reason we age.

Reactive Oxygen Species, or Free Radicals

Mitochondria produce unstable molecules called free radicals as a by-product of energy production. A relatively new name for free radicals is *reactive oxygen species,* or ROS. Reactive oxygen species are unstable because they give up an electron to the oxidative process. Because nature abhors instability, the free radical tries to steal an electron from another molecule, producing another free radical, which in turn steals an electron, and so forth. In this manner, the production of free radicals is a continuous process that leads to aging and, ultimately, death. When ROS build up in cells, the result is *oxidative stress,* a continual struggle between the forces that cause oxidative damage and those that protect against it.

Energy production in the mitochondria is a prime source of ROS, but not the only one. Glycation bonds, where glucose molecules attach themselves to proteins, are virtual free-radical factories. Excessive psychological stress, environmental toxins, and chronically inflamed tissues often trigger free-radical production.

Normally, our cells have effective defense mechanisms to protect us from the damage of oxidative stress. The enzymes superoxide dismutase (SOD) and catalase turn antioxidants into harmless oxygen and water. Given proper nourishment, our cells produce antioxidant compounds that induce ROS-overwhelmed cells to commit suicide. Phagocytes, which are debris-eating immune system cells, dispose of the dead cells in much the same way that crows and other carrion-eating animals dispose of roadkill. If we didn't ask too much of these inborn cleanup mechanisms, we would look younger and our lives would be longer. Instead, we place great demands on our endogenous antioxidants with diets high in starches, sugars, and foods cooked over high heat; constant exposure to airborne environmental poisons; and by living with psychological stress instead of learning to control how we react to it. Thus we overwhelm the normal process of *apoptosis,* in which cells complete their life cycle and die, with an overabundance of reactive oxygen species.

Oxidative Stress and Illness

As we age, our built-in antioxidant mechanisms lose their effectiveness, leaving the pathways open to various forms of damage. ROS play an important role in many degenerative and chronic diseases because of the damage free radicals do to DNA. Diabetes, heart and vascular disorders, Alzheimer's disease, rheumatoid arthritis and other autoimmune conditions, chronic fatigue, macular degeneration, and kidney disease are among the most prominent consequences of long-term oxidative stress. Oxidative damage that leads to the death of nerve-protecting tissues is probably the basic mechanism in neurological diseases of all sorts, including conditions ranging from multiple sclerosis to dementia. Unrepaired, oxidative DNA damage can lead to cell mutation, turning the cells into malignant tumors. Additionally, oxidative stress reduces the production and efficacy of acetylcholine, the brain chemical responsible for cognition, muscular strength, and coordination. Finally, oxidative stress increases the activity of NF-κB, decreasing the rate of death among exhausted cells and increasing the likelihood of tumor growth.

SNPs and Oxidative Stress

Individuals vary greatly in their susceptibility to ROS damage in different tissues. SNPs (single nucleotide polymorphisms) may explain the tendency often seen in families to get one disease or another. For example, studies have uncovered a variation in the enzyme manganese superoxide dismutase that is linked to increased risk of breast cancer in some premenopausal women. This discovery led researchers to examine the diets of women with this particular SNP. They found that women whose diets were high in antioxidant-rich foods were far less likely to develop breast cancer than those who consumed lower amounts of dietary antioxidants. The molecular mechanisms linking various SNPs to dietary interventions is the subject of much current research.

METHYLATION

Another area of considerable research activity is methylation. That is the process whereby certain genes are activated and others are deactivated during one's lifetime. DNA is composed of strings of nucleotides grouped into genes. Most genes in our DNA are active during embryonic development, when we grow from a single fertilized cell to a tiny mass of undifferentiated cells, and then become a fetus in which cells are differentiated into all the tissues that comprise a human being. When a gene is no longer needed, it is turned off. Many genes are silenced at birth, and the trend accelerates, especially after age twenty-five, with increasing numbers of genes being turned off as we age. The silencing of genes is thought to be one of the major factors in aging and ultimately death. Yet DNA methylation is essential for normal cell development and function.

The process begins when one carbon atom and three hydrogen atoms link to form a methyl group and attach themselves to a gene. When this happens, the methyl group generates a chromatin structure known as decondensed DNA. (Chromatin is the Slinky toy–like structure that protects DNA from damage.) Decondensed DNA turns off the gene transcription machinery so that encoded proteins cannot be synthesized. This prevents the creation of unnecessary proteins. An important example of this phenomenon is that one of the two X chromosomes in female mammals, including human beings, is inactivated by methylation.

Sometimes methyl groups attach to the wrong genes and ignore the correct ones. The result is detrimental increases or decreases in gene activity, with needed proteins not being synthesized and others being created unnecessarily. In the worst possible case, methylation may turn off tumor suppressor genes, allowing cancer to develop. Controlling methylation is beginning to be recognized as a crucial part of aging management. One factor already identified that helps optimize methylation is decreasing blood levels of the adrenal stress hormone cortisol. High levels of serum cortisol interfere with the efficiency of the methylation process.

INTRICATE WEB OF CAUSE AND EFFECT

Glycation, inflammation, oxidation, and methylation—the four factors in the aging equation—form an intricate web of cause and effect. Each feeds and is fed by the others. All four factors are present in even the healthiest people. When they get out of control, the principal culprits are improper nutrition and excessive stress, both physical and psychological. Since the way we eat and the way we handle stress are largely matters of personal choice, it is within our power to minimize the ill effects of these four processes. The next chapter explains how we can harness hormones, the body's chemical messengers, to work in the service of our anti-aging goals.

CHAPTER 5

Glands, Hormones, and Their Effect on Aging

IT IS BY LOGIC THAT WE PROVE,
BUT BY INTUITION THAT WE DISCOVER.
—*Henri Poincaré*

Aging management depends on more than minimizing DNA damage and optimizing DNA repair, important as these goals are. Maintaining and improving the way hormones, the body's chemical messengers, function is another important objective. The human body's intricate hormone system evolved over a million years as a means of communication from cell to cell. Hormones are responsible for maintaining balance among organ systems as diverse as the brain, immune system, and gastrointestinal tract.

The cascade of events triggered by the release of a hormone begins in the hypothalamus of the brain. The signal that stimulates a hormone's release may be a thought, an emotion, or a change in the immediate environment. Everything that happens at the cellular level originates in the brain. That is why the brain's health is so crucial to general health and well-being. With optimal hormonal levels, mental, sexual, and physiological performance is optimized; bone density and body composition are improved, and the body is in balance.

Hormonal levels decline as we age, and are directly related to changes in body shape, body composition, and skin quality. These are only the visible changes caused by hormonal decline. More important are the internal changes that predispose people to age-related degenerative ailments such as cardiovascular disease, diabetes, Alzheimer's disease, and cancer. The aging process results in the loss of elasticity in muscles and skin but it also reduces the capacity of the capillaries, the tiniest of blood vessels, and impairs their ability to bring hormones to tissues where they are needed. The fact that inadequate nutrition and excessive stress have a negative impact on hormonal levels completes the list of obstacles we must address if we are to maintain optimal health as we age.

COMMUNICATION AND HOMEOSTASIS

The keys to understanding how hormones act are the related concepts of communication and *homeostasis*. The hormonal signal originates with the release of prehormones by the hypothalamus to receptors in other parts of the brain, continues from there to the glands, and then to the trillions of cells in the body. Hormones interact with receptors on the cell membrane, stimulating the membrane to circulate messages within the cells through structures known as *second messenger complexes*. Hormones interact with DNA using these chemical and electromagnetic intermedi-

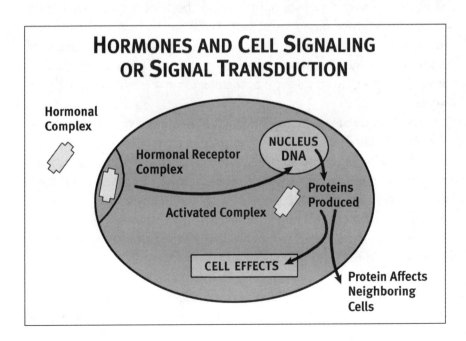

HORMONES AND CELL SIGNALING OR SIGNAL TRANSDUCTION

Hormonal Complex

Hormonal Receptor Complex

NUCLEUS DNA

Activated Complex

Proteins Produced

CELL EFFECTS

Protein Affects Neighboring Cells

aries, signaling genes to do their work. The chemical equivalent of a "mission accomplished" message provides feedback to the brain through series of additional hormonal messengers. All this occurs within seconds, or less.

The hormonal feedback loop is a crucial component in keeping the body in a state of equilibrium, or homeostasis. We may crave mental or emotional stimulation at times—some of us more often than others—but our body's prime desire is for balance. This balance is provided by the signaling power of our hormones, carrying messages among our organs that say, in effect, "Let's have a little more of this, a little less of that. OK, that's good, now keep it that way."

A good example of this drive for homeostasis is found in the actions of insulin and *glucagon*. Insulin is the hormone that carries glucose to the cells and tucks it away in the form of *glycogen* for the mitochondria to use to produce energy. Glycogen is also stored in the liver as a backup in case the mitochondria seem about to run out of raw materials. Since insulin's job is to lower blood sugar by sending glucose into storage, it would defeat its own purpose by sending out orders to the liver to release sugar into the blood. That's what glucagon does. Both insulin and glucagon take their cues from the hypothalamus to provide the proper balance of saving and spending blood sugar for energy.

A similar hormonal balancing occurs between the hormones epinephrine (also known as adrenaline) and insulin in times of acute stress. We all know the "fight or flight" reaction that occurs when something startles or frightens us. The instant the brain perceives danger, it signals the adrenal glands, located on the kidneys (hence the name, ad-renal), to flood the bloodstream with epinephrine, which performs a number of functions in a flash. It mobilizes the glycogen stored in your liver, causing your blood sugar to rise. Your reflexes sharpen, your mental clarity soars, and your muscles receive a surge of energy. The smooth muscles that line your blood vessels contract to reduce the tendency to bleed, and there is an increase in the chemicals that cause blood to clot. Meanwhile, because you need to protect your brain from an overload of sugar, your pancreas releases some extra insulin, pushing additional glucose into your muscle cells for added energy. These are but two of the ways that hormones protect us and work to preserve balance in our bodies.

Nothing happens in isolation in the body. Hormones strive to maintain the balance among organ systems, and the brain strives to maintain the balance among hormones. If an organ is sick or damaged, the balance of hormones is disturbed. If something in the body's environment disturbs the balance of hormones, such as poor nutrition or excessive stress, organ sickness or damage is likely to result. When we are young, maintaining homeostasis is less of an issue than it is by the time we reach middle age. We are born with a good supply of *functional organ reserve,* the capacity to mobilize defenses that enable us to withstand infection, environmental stress, or abuse, and maintain optimal health and functionality of our organ systems.

In our twenties, we have between 300 and 400 percent of the functional organ reserve necessary to maintain physiological health. The reserve drops to about 150 percent in middle age and to less than 100 percent when we reach our sixties and later. The more we can do to maintain organ reserve, the more we will be able to handle the aging process and the stresses of the increasingly toxic environment in which we find ourselves in the twenty-first century.

Emotional stress increasingly takes its toll on us as we age. Research has disclosed that many of the same hormones found in the brain exist in the gastrointestinal tract and the immune system. Another series of studies has established the connection between elevated levels of the adrenal stress hormones and suppressed immune function. These discoveries reinforce the link between body wellness and mental health that has spawned the new field of psychoneuroimmunology.

The degree of physical and mental equilibrium we maintain determines our level of health and how we age. This equation works in both directions: our balance affects our health, and our health affects our balance. Each plays a crucial role in the process of aging.

HOW AGING AFFECTS HORMONES

A brief look at how hormone signals are transmitted to the cells helps explain how aging affects our body's response to these signals. Each hormone molecule hitches a ride on a molecule called a *carrier protein* and travels through the circulatory system to its destination on a particular cell. The hormone then sheds its carrier and docks with a receptor site on the cell membrane. The receptor site is shaped to accommodate the hormone, much as a jigsaw puzzle piece is shaped to fit together with other pieces. The connection is not only three-dimensional, it is also maintained by electrostatic and electromagnetic interaction between the cell membrane and the hormone molecule. Once the hormone is docked, the cell membrane activates a series of second messenger complexes, which either enter the cell itself to activate or repress target genes or activate another complex already within the cell to carry out the same mission. The affected genes respond by synthesizing enzymes to perform specific functions or by remaining inactive, depending on the instructions relayed to the hormone by the second messengers. The enzymes may also cross the cell membrane and affect neighboring cells. That is how communication occurs both within and between cells and how homeostasis is maintained or restored.

Cell membranes are composed of omega-3 and omega-6 fatty acids. You get these fatty acids from food. If your diet is poor in either type of fatty acid, the receptor—the cell's docking station—on the cell membrane is apt to become distorted and inflexible, resulting in the hormone interaction being blunted or failing to occur. Further, the quality and quantity of the second messengers determine the strength of the signal received in the cell. One class of second messengers amplifies the hormone's signal; another class dampens it. If the second messengers are strong and present in the proper proportion, just a small amount of the hormone will deliver the desired effect. If, however, the level of second messengers is low or the ratio among them is out of balance, then the hormone level may be insufficient to evoke a response in the cell.

Aging affects every step in the cell-signaling process—the quantity and quality of the hormones, the sensitivity of receptors on the cell membrane, and the quantity and quality of the second messengers. As we grow older, genes are increasingly deactivated. Some of these are the genes that control synthesis of various hormones. Others control the metabolism of fatty acids. Thus, as our supply of hormones diminishes, so does our supply of the substances that keep our cell membranes sufficiently flexible to accommodate the shape of the hormones seeking to attach to cell receptors. Glycation may also play a role here. When sugar molecules attach to proteins—remember that hormones are proteins—the molecules are deformed and no longer fit their receptors. Additionally, the presence of undue physical or emotional stress and its resulting elevation of cortisol has a negative impact on the levels of other hormones.

Some of this deterioration of the cell-signaling process is inevitable as we age. But there is ample clinical and empirical evidence that we can slow the aging process and live healthier, longer lives than conventional wisdom would suggest is possible.

GLANDS

A gland is a group of cells that manufactures and discharges a hormone to be used in some part of the body. Glands can be classified as *merocrine, apocrine,* or *holocrine,* depending on how the secretion is accomplished, and as *endocrine* or *exocrine,* depending on how their secretions are carried to the place where they do their work. In merocrine glands, the secretion forms within cells and is passed through the cell membranes into secretory ducts. In apocrine glands, such as the mammary glands, the secretion forms in the ends of cells, which break off and become part of the secretion. Holocrine glands secrete entire cells and their contents. The oil (sebaceous) glands in the skin are holocrine glands.

Exocrine glands contain ducts that carry their secretions to a body surface such as the skin or mucous membranes. The sebaceous and salivary glands are exocrine glands. Endocrine glands have no ducts; they deliver their secretions directly into the blood or lymph. These are the glands that concern us as we take a tour of the endocrine system. Then we'll look more deeply at the actions of the endocrine hormones most involved in aging and its management.

The Hypothalamus

The hypothalamus is the endocrine system's master control center. A part of the brain, the hypothalamus receives information from nerves about the internal condition of the body and about the external environment. It then responds to this information by sending signals to appropriate nerves or glands. Among the body functions the hypothalamus controls as part of its hormone-signaling activities are maintenance of water balance, metabolism of sugar and fat, and regulation of body temperature.

The Pituitary Gland

Located just below the hypothalamus is the tiny pituitary gland, which is divided into two sections called the anterior lobe and the posterior lobe. The pituitary controls many bodily processes, including growth, reproduction, and metabolism. Each lobe of the pituitary has its own distinct role. The anterior lobe secretes human growth hormone (HGH), which promotes the growth and maintenance of muscle and bone and plays a crucial role in how we age. The anterior lobe also secretes a variety of hormones that simulate other glands, earning the pituitary the title of the body's master gland. The posterior lobe releases oxytocin, which specifically targets the smooth muscle of the uterus, controlling its tone and ability to contract. It also provides vasopressin, which controls the contraction of the smooth muscle of blood vessels, and antidiuretic hormone, which prevents excessive loss of water through the kidneys. Evidence suggests that the pituitary hormones are actually secreted in the hypothalamus and sent to the pituitary, where they are stored and released as needed.

The Thyroid Gland

The thyroid gland is located in the neck, just below the larynx. It produces and secretes two hormones, thyroxine (T4) and triiodothyronine (T3), which control the body's rate of metabolism. Both these hormones regulate the speed at which body cells burn carbohydrates and fats to produce energy. T3 and T4 are also important in the development of bones and nerve cells and help maintain normal heart rate and blood pressure, as well as digestive and reproductive functions.

The Adrenal Glands

The two adrenal glands sit like caps on top of the kidneys. Each gland contains two parts, the outer cortex and the inner medulla. During gestation, the cortex comes from a part of the developing embryo that gives rise to the sex organs. The medulla arises from a part that also develops into the sympathetic nervous system, the part of the nervous system that controls muscles not under our conscious control. Among its other functions, the adrenal cortex secretes the corticosteroid hormones, including cortisol, which will be discussed in more detail shortly. The adrenal medulla mobilizes the body's stress response by producing epinephrine, also known as adrenaline, and norepinephrine, two hormones that initiate the fight-or-flight response. These hormones prepare the body for immediate action by increasing heart rate, blood pressure, metabolism, and blood glucose levels and by boosting the blood supply to the muscles.

The Pancreas

The pancreas, which is located behind the stomach, produces the hormones insulin and glucagon, which control the level of glucose in the blood. The pancreas also provides enzymes essential to digestion.

The Ovaries and Testes

The ovaries and testes are, respectively, the female and male endocrine glands. Ovaries secrete the hormones estrogen and progesterone, which control the development of female secondary sex characteristics, including breasts and added body fat around the hips and thighs. They also regulate menstruation. Testes produce hormones called androgens, including testosterone, which is responsible for the development of male secondary sex characteristics, including increased facial hair and lowered voice pitch. Estrogen and testosterone are present in people of both sexes, just in different concentrations.

The Pineal Gland

Deep within the brain is a very small endocrine gland called the pineal, which produces and secretes melatonin. This hormone has several functions, including regulation of the body's clock and its sleep-wake cycle.

The Thymus Gland

The thymus gland, located in the chest cavity in front of and just above the heart, controls the immune system by providing immune system cells known as lymphocytes, or T cells. These secretions are important in defending the cells against bacteria, viruses, and other invaders by producing antibodies and phagocytes. The thymus gland grows rapidly during the first two years of life and reaches its maximum size at puberty. It shrinks as we age, with a resulting decline in immune system function.

HORMONES ASSOCIATED WITH AGING

Aging affects all steps in the process of cell-to-cell communication. Advancing age is linked to hormone imbalance, declining receptor sensitivity, and an imbalance of second messengers within cells. Changes on the cellular level in turn affect tissue and organ systems throughout the body, causing many of the more obvious signs and symptoms of aging. When hormone levels are consistently too high or too low, homeostasis is compromised. This section explores the main hormones associated with aging to further explain how hormone imbalance affects health.

It is common to speak of male-specific and female-specific hormones, but both types of hormones are found in both sexes. What differs is which hormones are dominant. Men have more of the androgen hormones (testosterone and androsterone) than the estrogen hormones (estradiol, estriol, and estrone) and women have more estrogens than androgens. Conditions that result from a disruption of the balance between male and female hormones are among the most emotionally painful imaginable. Fortunately, such conditions are rare and can often be reversed through medical intervention.

The Androgenic Hormones

The male hormones, collectively called androgen hormones or the androgenic hormones, are secreted by the Leydig cells in the testes as the result of stimulation by two pituitary hormones, follicle-stimulating hormone (FSH) and luteinizing hormone (LH). The primary and best known of the androgen hormones is testosterone. Androgens control the development and maintenance of masculine characteristics—the male sex organs, secondary sex characteristics, and personality features. A subset of the androgens is secreted by the adrenal cortex. Chief among the adrenal androgens is DHEA, which will be discussed separately.

Free testosterone, which makes up 2 to 3 percent of the total testicular secretion, is the active form of the hormone, and is responsible for shaping both the male physique and mentality. Testosterone contributes to libido and supports the ability to maintain and build muscles and burn fat. It is essential in supporting optimal skin tone, bone strength, immunity, and a healthy emotional state. Testosterone deficiencies are directly related to low sex drive and mental depression. Sparse facial hair, slow beard growth, and diminished body hair are commonly related to deficiencies in this hormone as well. The inability to build muscle, maintain bone mass, and burn fat are often related to testosterone insufficiency. Osteoporosis, anemia, and unstable emotions coupled with indecisiveness are also related to deficiencies in testosterone. Excess testosterone results in an overactive libido, an overabundance of body hair, reduced scalp hair, and excessively aggressive behavior. Greasy, oily skin and acne are other telltale signs of excessive testosterone levels.

An enzyme system called *aromatase* is active within the body, mainly in fat cells. Aromatase converts a portion of testosterone into the estrogen hormones. In men, estrogen stimulates the production *of sex steroid-binding globulin* (SSBG), a limiting factor that binds with testosterone, restricting the amount of free testosterone available. The greater the amount of SSBG secreted, the more testosterone is removed from the circulatory system. This leads to weight gain, particularly in the abdomen and around the waist. Since this body fat configuration is also associated with insulin resistance, there is reason to believe that the decline in testosterone commonly seen in middle age is related to the glycation process that renders insulin less effective as we age.

Other androgens include androstanediol, which is thought to act as the main regulator of sex-hormone secretions; androsterone, which is present in roughly the same amounts in men and women; and androstenedione, which is produced by both the testes and ovaries and is converted to both testosterone and estrone, one of the estrogen hormones. Androstenedione is noted for its body-building abilities. Its use as a supplement has been banned by the International Olympic Committee.

The 5a-reductase enzyme system converts some testosterone into 5-dihydrotestosterone (DHT), which binds to the same receptor sites as testosterone, further decreasing the effectiveness of whatever free testosterone is available. Production of DHT increases with age. It is related to hair loss, prostate enlargement, and the consequent difficulties with urination that many men experience beginning in middle age.

Among lean young men, the ratio of testosterone to estrogen is approximately 50:1. Aging decreases that ratio. The speed of the decline is related to both genetic and environmental factors. By middle age, the ratio drops to about 20:1. The high energy and assertive behavior common among men of high-school and college age mellows into something more passive and tolerant. Fortunately a 20:1 ratio is still sufficient to maintain vibrant good health and an excellent quality of life.

Changes in body composition and male personality characteristics are increasingly recognized as *andropause,* the male equivalent of female menopause. As aging proceeds, testosterone-to-estrogen ratios drop to approximately 8:1, bringing about still more fatty deposits in the abdomen, as well as accelerating loss of muscle mass and bone. That some men find themselves becoming lethargic and lacking in physical and mental energy is another reason to associate the decline in testosterone with insulin resistance.

In addition to the lifestyle changes that will be suggested in Chapter 6 in relation to managing insulin resistance, men troubled by declining testosterone-to-estrogen ratios should note that even moderate intake of alcoholic beverages has been associated with increased estrogen levels in the blood. Alcohol decreases liver enzymes that break down estrogen for excretion, resulting in a buildup of estrogen in the bloodstream. A deficiency in zinc has also been found to be related to an increase in the aromatase enzyme system, which turns testosterone into estrogen.

The Estrogen Hormones

The ovaries produce most of the female hormones, synthesizing them from the androgenic hormones through the action of enzymes. Some estrogens are also produced in the adrenal glands and the breasts, especially in postmenopausal women. The three estrogens are estradiol, estriol, and estrone. Estradiol is produced from testosterone. Estrone is produced from androstenedione and is weaker than estradiol. Before menopause, estradiol is dominant, but after menopause the proportions are reversed. The estrogens are responsible for the development of female secondary sex characteristics and are involved in controlling ovulation and the menstrual cycle, which is why most birth control pills contain estrogens. They are also related to the synthesis of collagen, brain function and memory, bone density, muscle and fat-cell metabolism, and blood fat levels.

Deficiencies in the three estrogens often result in wrinkled skin due to the hormones' connection to collagen. Postmenopausal women are susceptible to bone loss, particularly in the weight-bearing bones of the pelvis and legs. Cognitive impairment and short-term memory loss can be a result of estrogen deficiencies in older women. The relationship between estrogen deficiency and low HDL and high LDL cholesterol levels is the main reason women are subject to higher rates of arteriosclerosis and heart attacks after menopause.

The distressing mood swings of menopause are a result of estrogen insufficiency. Hot flashes can be caused by either too much or too little estrogen. Excessive estrogen production can manifest itself as painful breasts, cysts and cystic masses, uterine fibroid tumors, and anxiety. Estrogen imbalances are also associated with water retention, bloating, and difficulty in losing weight.

An excess of estradiol and estrone has been linked to an overgrowth of breast, uterine, and ovarian tissues, which may result in cancer. Estriol, on the other hand, has been called the protective estrogen because it seems to inhibit the proliferative effects of the other two estrogen components. Levels of the three estrogen hormones can be determined by tests of blood or saliva.

Progesterone is another female sex hormone, produced by the corpus luteum within the ovary following ovulation. It is also produced in small amounts in the adrenals by the conversion from pregnenolone. Levels of progesterone start to decline at age thirty-five. Women who do not ovulate produce insufficient progesterone. Progesterone's main function is a supportive role during the phase of the menstrual cycle between ovulation and the onset of the menses. It helps prepare the lining of the uterus for implantation of a fertilized egg.

Progesterone joins estriol in its anticancer effects and plays an important role in damping the proliferative effect of estradiol and estrone on the breast, uterus, and ovaries. Progesterone counterbalances the estrogens' water-retention effects and supports the building of new bone tissue. It has a calming effect on the brain, enhancing sleep and counteracting the anxiety-producing effects of the estrogens. It has anti-inflammatory qualities and supports the myelin coating that protects nerve fibers in the peripheral nervous system.

Deficiencies in progesterone can result in water retention, weight gain, bone loss, anxiety, sleep problems, painful breasts, and shorter menstrual cycles. Heavy menstrual bleeding is also common. Flare-ups of arthritis or a general inflammatory state are also frequently associated with a deficiency of progesterone. High progesterone levels can result in dizziness, sleepiness, and nausea. Excess progesterone may be converted to cortisol, which is associated with rapid aging. Polycystic ovarian syndrome (PCOS), one of the symptom sets associated with insulin resistance, is characterized by obesity, excessive facial hair, and lack of ovulation and menstruation; all these signs and symptoms are also related to a surplus of progesterone, some of which has turned into testosterone.

Hormones Equally Prevalent in Both Sexes

The respective balances of the androgenic and estrogenic hormones are what differentiate men and women. Variations in hormone balance within individuals give them the personality traits and physical characteristics that make them seem more masculine or feminine. With the exception of DHEA, which is discussed first, the rest of the hormones most associated with aging affect both sexes in roughly the same manner.

DHEA

DHEA is produced in the adrenal glands from the precursor molecule pregnenolone, which is synthesized from cholesterol. Remember this fact when you hear the common myth that all cholesterol is evil. If we managed to remove all cholesterol from our bodies, not only would we be unable to synthesize any sex hormones, but we also would dissolve because cholesterol is a significant component of cell membranes. Fortunately, we cannot eliminate cholesterol from our bodies because the liver manufactures most of it, regardless of how little dietary fat we consume.

However, it is possible to be deficient in cholesterol, throwing our hormones out of balance.

DHEA's main function is to serve as a precursor to testosterone in both men and women. In addition, DHEA has been shown to augment the efficiency of the immune system. It is also related to the ratio of lean muscle to fat tissue. Furthermore, it has been shown to help maintain optimal brain function.

In men, deficiencies of DHEA have been directly related to poor immunity, psychological depression, low metabolic rates, low estrogen levels (because testosterone produces estrogen), and low HDL ("good") cholesterol levels. Low levels of HDL cholesterol are known to be related to an increased risk of cardiovascular disease. Excessively high DHEA levels in men have been related to high estrogen levels, especially estradiol. In women DHEA deficiency can result in low libido, poor immunity, depression, and a low metabolic rate, resulting in weight gain. In excess, symptoms of masculinization occur, including excess acne, greasy skin, loss of scalp hair, facial hair growth, and excessive libido.

DHEA is the most abundant of the steroid hormones. Its production peaks in early adulthood and declines as we age.

Melatonin

Melatonin (Greek for "night worker") is produced by the pineal gland, whose function aside from melatonin production is relatively unknown. It is suppressed during the day by light, and its secretion is stimulated by darkness. It collaborates with cortisol in controlling the daily (circadian) rhythms of sleeping and wakefulness: melatonin is dominant in the nighttime, helping us fall asleep, and cortisol peaks in the early morning hours, stimulating us to awaken. Melatonin influences production of many of the sex hormones. Melatonin receptors are found on the ovaries and high doses of melatonin have been tested for use in birth control in women. The hormone also seems to influence the secretion of thyroid hormones. Additionally, melatonin is a potent antioxidant and thus a protector of DNA from free-radical damage.

Melatonin deficiency is usually manifested by symptoms that include trouble falling asleep and restless sleep in general. Symptoms of too much melatonin include difficulty awakening—possibly because in excess melatonin dampens the wakening effects of cortisol—and unpleasantly vivid dreams. Melatonin has been found to be suspiciously lacking in adequate levels in breast cancer patients. Cancer patients who undergo chemotherapy or radiation therapy as their initial treatment have been found to have a better long-term prognosis if they take melatonin supplements.

The Thyroid Hormones

The thyroid hormones consist of thyrotropin (thyroid-stimulating hormone or TSH), thyroxine (T4), and triiodothyronine (T3). TSH is produced by the pituitary and stimulates the thyroid gland to produce T4. The liver and other tissues convert T4 to T3, the most active of the thyroid hormones. The amino acid tyrosine is a precursor to T4; selenium helps convert T4 to T3. These two nutrients are essential to healthy thyroid function. Iodine, a nonmetallic element, is another important nutrient involved in the function of the thyroid gland. A lack of iodine is a cause of deficiency in the thyroid hormones, which is why table salt is iodized.

The thyroid hormones have several functions. They regulate the entry of oxygen into the cells, controlling most physiological processes, including basal metabolic rate, body temperature, ovulation, heart rate, brain activity, skin health, and hair growth. Thyroid hormone deficiency usually results in a low metabolic rate, weight gain, low body temperature, cold hands and feet, grogginess and muscular stiffness in the morning, constipation, and dry and brittle skin and hair. Menstrual irregularities and lack of ovulation are common in women with underactive thyroid glands. The inability to perspire and an enlarged thyroid gland (goiter) are also common signs of thyroid deficiency. Excess thyroid hormone, especially T3, can produce heart palpitations, disordered sleep, nervousness and agitation, and bulging eyes.

Human Growth Hormone

Human growth hormone (HGH or somatotropin) has long been the major focus of longevity journals, touted as the Fountain of Youth and the key component of any anti-aging program. These claims could hardly be further from the truth. Although high HGH levels are essential during adolescence, its concentration in the body drops drastically in the early twenties and continues to decline throughout life. Still, it is important to health and well-being as we age.

The growth-hormone production cycle begins with growth-hormone-releasing hormone (GHRH), which is manufactured within the hypothalamus. True to its name, GHRH stimulates production and release of somatotropin from the pituitary gland. Grehlin, which is produced by specific cells in the digestive tract, also stimulates HGH. Somatostatin inhibits the release of HGH and is also produced in the hypothalamus. Since the hypothalamus produces both the stimulant and the inhibitor of HGH release, it acts as the controlling factor through one of the body's elegant feedback loops.

Human growth hormone by itself has a direct effect on tissues and organs, including muscle, brain, skin, and bone, and on immune function. In excess it can also be converted within the liver into a more potent and active form, called insulinlike growth factor (IGF-1). An overabundance of insulin in the blood, the consequence of insulin resistance, is the most common trigger of IGF-1. This hormone has been found to be a risk factor for several kinds of cancer.

HGH's primary role is to increase anabolic activity, which builds lean tissue—more muscle, denser bones, and thicker skin. HGH is also associated with increased fat burning. It improves brain function as well as overall immune function. It carries off lactic acid, which is generated in the muscles whenever we move and causes the muscle aches so familiar to weekend athletes. HGH also repairs the microscopic damage to muscles that is the inevitable result of motion.

Eighty percent of growth hormone is generated during slow-wave (deep) sleep, particularly between the hours of 11 p.m. and 1 a.m., assuming melatonin is doing its job of setting the body's clock. The other 20 percent is secreted during and just after vigorous exercise. People who suffer from insomnia, and those who live sedentary lives, are apt to be deficient in growth hormone. It has been found that growth hormone is deficient in people who have fibromyalgia, probably because a prime component of the fibromyalgia syndrome is dysfunctional sleep.

Symptoms of growth-hormone deficiency include musculoskeletal pain, muscle and joint weakness, thin skin, increased body fat, poor bone density or osteoporosis, poor memory, and impaired immune function. Excess growth-hormone secretion is associated with acromegaly, a chronic disease that occurs in middle age. Acromegaly is characterized by elongation of the bones of the arms and legs and enlargement of some bones in the head, edema, joint pain, dizziness, and an increase in soft tissues, including swelling of the tongue. An overabundance of HGH is often accompanied by a decrease in apoptosis, the natural process in which cells die and are carried away in excretion. Inhibited apoptosis is linked to cancer. An increase in inflammatory cytokines and leukotrienes is another byproduct of excess HGH. Fortunately, excess HGH is uncommon, unless you buy and take one of the HGH products so widely advertised. Careful medical supervision is a must when dealing with a growth-hormone deficiency.

Cortisol

As vital as it is to human life and function, cortisol has been dubbed the age-accelerating hormone. It is produced by the adrenal glands in response to adrenocorticotropic hormone (ACTH), which is released by the pituitary in response to another hormone—corticotropin-releasing hormone (CRH)—from the hypothalamus. Cortisol has an anti-inflammatory effect (another name for it is cortisone, which is also the name of a trademarked pharmaceutical drug). To ensure a steady supply of energy, cortisol helps break down glycogen (the stored form of glucose) upon its release by the liver and cells, and it helps break down fats and proteins. It is part of the backup system that ensures a supply of glucose to those parts of the brain that cannot function without it.

That's the good news. The bad news about cortisol is that stress increases it, as part of the body's protective mechanism. Chronic stress leads to chronically elevated cortisol levels, which are common in middle age. Elevated cortisol is related to a breakdown of collagen and elastin in skin (causing wrinkles) and in joint, bone, and muscle tissue (causing aches and pains). Elevated cortisol has a major inhibiting effect on sex hormones, thyroid hormones, growth hormone, and DHEA. High levels of cortisol have been shown to damage neurons of the central nervous system, causing memory loss. Relatively new research has documented damage to cortisol receptors in the hypothalamus, resulting in further elevation of cortisol due to poor feedback receptivity. Chronic cortisol elevations cause damage in both thymic and lymphatic tissues, decreasing the immune function. Clinical depression occurs as a result of a decrease in some brain chemicals that is related to elevated cortisol.

Even though cortisol is an effective anti-inflammatory, chronic high levels increase formation of bad (inflammatory) eicosanoids and decrease good (anti-inflammatory) eicosanoids. Finally, elevated cortisol interferes with the second messengers that help transmit hormone signals within the cells. For all these reasons, the designation of cortisol as an accelerator of aging could not be more appropriate.

Cortisol deficiency can result in sugar cravings and reactive hypoglycemia, the condition in which insulin resistance causes a roller-coaster blood sugar effect after a meal or snack high in sugars and starches. Dizziness, mental confusion, and fatigue are all features of reactive hypoglycemia. Simple ways to decrease cortisol include age-management programs and stress-relaxation methods.

Leptin

Only recently identified, leptin is produced by fat cells. One of its functions is to inhibit somatostatin, reducing its effect in suppressing HGH. Leptin has been linked to obesity, in that it is overabundant in proportion to the surplus of fat cells. People who are underweight are usually leptin deficient. The current theory is that leptin provides the signal that it's time to stop eating and get moving. The paradox that leptin levels are high in obese people even though it is the signal to stop eating is probably solved by an analogy to insulin resistance. People who are seriously overweight often report that they cannot tell when they have had enough to eat. It is likely that glycation, which causes insulin resistance, also causes leptin resistance. Glucose molecules attach themselves to leptin molecules, making it impossible for the leptin receptors on cells to accept the message that it's time to stop eating.

THE IMPORTANCE OF HORMONE BALANCE

It is impossible to overstate the importance of hormone balance when it comes to aging management and the quest for a long and healthy life. Understanding the mechanisms and feedback loops of the various hormones will stand you in good stead in the next chapter, which deals with ways to influence and balance hormone levels.

CHAPTER 6

Diet, Exercise, and Aging

EVERY MAN TAKES THE LIMITS OF HIS OWN FIELD OF VISION
FOR THE LIMITS OF THE WORLD.

—*Arthur Schopenhauer*

Even more than baseball, eating is the all-American pastime. Food is part of virtually every human interaction. When we visit friends, they offer us food and we eat. We eat at weddings and funerals, parties and business meetings, sports events and the movies. We eat because food is available, not necessarily because we are hungry. We eat to be polite. We eat, and all but the fortunate few grow fat.

We have forgotten what every infant is born knowing: the single valid purpose of eating is to sustain life. Food is fuel for our cells, nothing more and nothing less. Real hunger is a signal from the brain that we are running low on fuel. Taking in food for any other reason is *recreational eating.*

Not only do we eat when we don't need to eat, but we also sit still far more than is good for us. We sit at a desk to work, drive to run an errand a half mile away, watch television from dinner to bedtime, park as close as possible to the door we wish to enter, and avoid stairs if an elevator is available. There are other, better, more life-extending ways to use our bodies, and some of them are fun.

This chapter is about diet and exercise, and the changes in lifestyle and habit that will slow the rate at which you age, no matter how many years you've already logged. It's about the things you can do, starting today, to give your genes the environment they need in which to serve you long and well. There is no physical condition that cannot be improved by a healthful diet or made worse by faulty nutrition. A sedentary lifestyle compounds the effects of poor nutrition. Here you will learn why this is true and what to do about it.

DIET AND AGING

You are what you eat, in the most literal sense. Ultimately, every molecule in your body is derived from the food you take in. What you eat controls which genes are expressed and which are inhibited. Genes produce enzymes, which catalyze the chemical processes that produce hormones, which control the functioning of your organs and tissues. What you eat is the primary determinant of how close you will come to realizing your genetic potential. The inevitable result of a poor diet is poor gene activation and early aging. By taking into your body only the foods that promote healthy aging, you accomplish three important objectives:

- Decreasing the amount of glucose in your blood and, hence, the occurrence of glycation.
- Optimizing the balance between insulin and glucagon.
- Maintaining an ideal pH level in your body fluids.

An anti-aging diet is different from a weight-loss diet in two important ways. First, in the anti-aging diet the emphasis is on altering body composition to a more youthful configuration, decreasing body fat and increasing muscle mass. Achieving this leads to an improvement in our ability to burn calories efficiently, getting the maximum benefit out of every bite of food we eat. Muscle burns calories at a higher rate than fat, and the resulting energy is closer to that of young people. Second, an anti-aging diet is not the kind of diet you go on for a fixed period of time and then forget about; it is a way of eating for the rest of your life.

By themselves, weight-loss diets almost never work. The statistics for people who lose significant amounts of weight and keep it off are dismal. More common than successful weight loss is the phenomenon of losing weight and then gaining it all back, and more. Evidence shows this kind of yo-yo dieting can be more harmful than being overweight to begin with. Here's why: Your body seeks homeostasis— keeping things the same— above all else. When you start losing weight, your body tries to keep things on an even keel. No matter how much you want to lose weight, your body reacts as though you are facing starvation. It slows down your metabolism to conserve energy. What you eat provides less energy and is more apt to be stored as fat. Also, if all you do is reduce your caloric intake without changing the composition of your diet, eventually you will start to lose muscle mass, which is exactly the opposite of what you want to achieve. Don't let this discourage you. You are about to learn how to design a way of eating that will help you lose weight if you want to, change your body shape in ways that will please you (and those around you), and provide you with more energy than you thought was possible.

Your genetic makeup has a great deal to say about whether and how you can lose weight. Some people seem to have an inherited characteristic that helps them store fat against times of famine. Our earliest ancestors got their food by hunting meat and picking nuts and berries, rather than by staying in one place and practicing agriculture. Some of us—at least 35 percent, and probably more—may have inherited what is known as the thrifty gene from them. The thrifty gene has yet to be identified in the human genome, but the theory is that this gene helped hunter-gatherers survive when the hunt was going badly. The thrifty gene may be the one that codes for the enzyme lipoprotein lipase (LPL), which is produced by fat cells and helps the body store energy as fat. Thus, if you have the thrifty gene, the more LPL your body produces, the more fat you store. The more your body perceives itself as facing starvation, the more LPL it will produce. This does not mean that you are doomed to obesity; it simply means that the dietary modifications recommended here are especially important to you.

No matter how highly motivated you are to achieve a life that is healthy, long, and full of energy, changing the way you eat is not a trivial task. It takes discipline to alter the habits of a lifetime. But the results come quickly, often within days, and are so striking—particularly with regard to increased energy and improved mood—that each day that passes makes it easier to stay with your plan. In addition, it is no harder to develop a good habit than a bad one. If you choose to change the way you eat, you can do it.

Balanced Nutrition

Nutritionists divide food into three categories called macronutrients: proteins, carbohydrates, and fats. During digestion, proteins mainly break down into amino acids, carbohydrates into sugars, and fats into fatty acids. Fats may be composed entirely of fatty substances, but few proteins or carbohydrates are purely protein or carbohydrate. We identify foods as protein or carbohydrate according to which macronutrient predominates.

Proteins are mainly animal products: meat, fish, poultry, eggs, and cheese. These proteins all contain fat to some extent, and even traces of carbohydrates. Vegetable proteins include soy and other legumes (beans) and nuts; these foods are higher in carbohydrates than are animal proteins. The amino acids in the proteins we eat combine to build the proteins— cells, tissues, enzymes, and hormones—of which our bodies are composed.

The conventional Western diet consists primarily of carbohydrates, which provide energy in the form of glucose. Carbohydrate foods include fruits, grains, and vegetables. Some carbohydrates are high in starch; others are not. Vegetables are often rich in fiber, which benefits the digestive system and reduces the absorption of fats.

Fatty acids are the essential components of all cell membranes and cell receptors, and are required in appropriate quantities to optimize hormonal signaling and hormonal responses both on the surface and within the cell. Fats slow down the digestion and absorption of carbohydrates, helping to keep blood sugar from rising too rapidly. Fats may be saturated or unsaturated. Unsaturated fats may be polyunsaturated or monounsaturated. Contrary to common belief, saturated fats are not the primary source of cholesterol, but they should be consumed in moderation because of their effect on the body's pH level. Vegetable oils (olive, corn, safflower, flaxseed, and primrose) are excellent sources of unsaturated fats. Monounsaturated fats come in two main types, omega-3 and omega-6, and are obtained as part of other foods or as nutritional supplements. They are not consumed as foods themselves. Both are important to good health, but most Americans consume too much of the omega-6 variety, which is especially plentiful in animal proteins. An imbalance of omega-3 and omega-6 fatty acids in which omega-6s predominate can give rise to inflammation.

Trans fats, or trans-fatty acids, are fats to avoid as much as possible. They inhibit the action of an enzyme that promotes production of the good eicosanoids, thus adding to the likelihood of chronic inflammation and autoimmune disease. Trans fats are manufactured; they do not occur in nature. They are listed on food labels as "partially hydrogenated vegetable oils," and are used in many processed foods, especially margarine and baked goods. Starting in 2006, a U.S. Food and Drug Administration regulation will require manufacturers to list trans fats on food-nutrition labels directly under the line for saturated fat.

In terms of energy, 1 gram of protein or carbohydrate yields 4 calories, while 1 gram of fat supplies 9 calories. With fat containing more than twice the energy of equal quantities of either protein or carbohydrate, an easy way to lose weight is to cut back on your intake of fat. However, eating processed low-fat foods is not the way to do that. To make low-fat food items palatable, manufacturers add large quantities of sugars (high fructose corn syrup, for example), with the unwanted consequence of raising your blood sugar and providing a rich source of the raw materials for glycation.

The rule of thumb for a beneficial balance of macronutrients is that 40 percent of your calories should come from carbohydrates and 30 percent each from proteins and fats. A 2,000-calorie intake works out this way:

Carbohydrates: 800 calories, 200 grams, or 21 ounces

Proteins: 600 calories, 150 grams, or 5.3 ounces

Fats: 600 calories, 66 grams, or 2.3 ounces

You can find the breakdown of macronutrients in the Nutrition Facts table on most packaged foods. *The Complete Book of Food Counts,* a book that provides this information for a huge variety of fresh, processed, and fast foods, is listed in Appendix C.

This combination of macronutrients differs considerably from the one recommended in the Food Pyramid published by the U.S. Department of Agriculture (USDA) and the American Dietetic Association, in which the target is 300 to 350 grams of carbohydrates. Since the USDA's guidelines determine the composition of meals served for school lunches and other

Cereal Grains and Autoimmune Diseases

Cereal grains—wheat, rye, barley, oats, corn, rice, sorghum, and millet—contain mainly starch and fiber, some protein, and in some cases traces of fat. Some of us descend from people who started eating grains 10,000 years ago, when the first tools for grinding grain were developed in the Middle East. Human beings cannot digest grains that are not ground because the nutrients in plant foods are enclosed within cells that our stomachs cannot break down. It took 5,000 years for the technology to grind grain to spread to northern Europe. It takes many thousands of years for human evolution to adapt to new environmental conditions. Actually, the human genome has undergone little change in the past 40,000 years. So, depending on your ancient heritage, you may be ill equipped to gain much nutritional benefit from eating grains, even the "whole" grains (grains ground without first milling off the outer coverings) that the USDA claims are good for you.

A current theory suggests that cereal grains may be one of the causes of autoimmune diseases such as rheumatoid arthritis and multiple sclerosis. If you suffer from an autoimmune disease, you may want to test this theory by eliminating all grain-based foods

group-meal sites that receive federal funding, these high-carbohydrate diets may be partially responsible for the so-called twin epidemics of obesity and diabetes that are currently rampant in the United States. Some people can metabolize this much glucose without difficulty, but the likelihood of that decreases with age and fades to zero in the presence of the thrifty gene.

People who are significantly overweight will need to trim their carbohydrate intake considerably, to 100 grams or less with corresponding increases in proteins and, to a lesser extent, fats. It is not unheard of for people who are insulin resistant to gain weight on a diet containing as few as 50 grams of carbohydrates. There is no way to know what is best for you except to experiment. When you find the right balance of proteins, carbohydrates, and fats you'll know it: your energy will soar, and if you are (breads, cereals, and the like) from your diet for a few months to see if it makes a difference in your health. Some people who have tried this have seen their autoimmune symptoms go into remission, or at least not get any worse.

The theory is that grains contain elements mimicking substances in the human body. When these elements get into the human blood-stream, immune system cells recognize them as foreign invaders and an autoimmune reaction ensues. Normally, the molecules that make up our food do not enter the bloodstream, but there are sit-uations—particularly in people whose diets are high in carbohy-drates—where the lining of the gut can become permeable, allowing molecules from partially digested foods to slip through. This condi-tion is known as *leaky gut syndrome*. It can cause vitamin and min-eral deficiencies, and if the theory of grain-induced autoimmunity holds true, leaky gut syndrome may contribute to the autoimmune diseases for which we presently have no other explanation. Evi-dence for this is found in the fact that autoimmune diseases are most common among people of northern European descent. Their incidence decreases as you trace the migration of agriculture diago-nally southeast to the Middle East, where grains were first ground and eaten.

overweight, your weight will decrease at a gratifying rate while your body fat redistributes itself in a pleasing way.

If you think you have the thrifty gene and are insulin resistant, you may well be wondering what carbohydrates you can eat and still gain the advantages of the anti-aging diet. The answer is to focus on leafy, high-fiber vegetables and members of the cabbage family—broccoli, cauli-flower, asparagus, kale, spinach, summer squashes, all kinds of lettuce, and other salad vegetables. Low-carbohydrate fruits include apples, all berries, melons, and citrus fruits. You will find a list of low-carbohydrate fruits and vegetables in Appendix A. When you count carbohydrates remember that you can deduct the fiber grams from the total. There is plenty to eat without turning to starchy vegetables such as potatoes, rice, corn, and winter squashes.

The Glycemic Index of Foods

The main reason to avoid foods with a high sugar content such as sweets, starches, low-fat foods, and many other processed foods is to keep your blood sugar as level as possible throughout the day. You want to keep your insulin level low, and to do that you need to ask the insulin-producing cells of your pancreas to do as little work as possible. A high-carbohydrate diet demands a great deal of insulin. When insulin is high, glucagon, the counterbalancing fat-burning hormone, is low. If you're interested in seeing how your blood sugar behaves during the day, you can buy a glucose monitor and check your blood sugar for a week or so. For a baseline, you should know your fasting blood sugar level, which is measured immediately upon waking up, before you have had anything to eat or drink. Normal fasting blood sugars range from 70 to 125. (The measurement is expressed as ml/dl—thousandths of a liter per 10 liters of blood.) A fasting blood sugar between 115 and 125 is grounds for suspicion of diabetes, and a reading above 125 first thing in the morning warns of impending or actual diabetes. It's also interesting to test just before you eat, immediately after eating, and one and two hours after a meal. If you wonder how a particular food will affect your blood sugar, testing before and one and two hours after you eat it will tell you what you need to know. There is no absolute rule about how high your blood sugar can go after a meal, but it should return to near-fasting level after two hours. What you don't want is a blood sugar level that behaves like a roller coaster. Insulin resistance, combined with a diet high in carbohydrates, makes that happen. The result is alternating surges of insulin and cortisol, first raising blood sugar and then bringing it down. You know about the aging effects of excess insulin and cortisol: that's the effect you are trying to avoid.

If your genetic makeup does not require you to minimize your carbohydrate intake, you should still know about the glycemic index of foods. This is a ranking of carbohydrate-containing foods on a scale from zero to 100 or above, according to the speed with which they get into the bloodstream and raise your blood sugar. Foods with a high index number cause blood sugar to soar. Low-index foods keep you on an even keel. The index was developed in the early 1980s as a way to help people with diabetes learn which foods cause the least fluctuation in their blood sugar levels.

Actually, there are two glycemic indexes: One measures the body's response to various carbohydrate-containing foods in comparison with carbohydrate in the form of 50 grams of glucose. The glucose response is given the value of 100. The glycemic index of other foods is expressed as a percentage of the glucose response. The second index uses 1 ounce of white bread as the standard, and foods are measured as a percentage of the response to white bread, which is 70 on the glucose scale. To convert the glycemic index of a food on the white-bread scale to the glucose scale, multiply the white-bread index by 1.43 (100 divided by 70, rounded up to two decimal places.) It doesn't matter which index you use, as long as you are consistent. So, if someone tells you the glycemic index of a food, you need to know what scale they are using. Foods with a glucose index of 70 or more are high-glycemic foods; they act quickly to raise blood sugar and trigger the insulin response you want to avoid. Foods with a glycemic index below 50 are slow-acting, low-glycemic foods, and those in the middle (50 to 69) are intermediate glycemic foods.

The fat content of a food item has a profound effect on its glycemic index. A bagel has a glycemic index on the glucose scale of 72. Spreading it with cream cheese, a fat, lowers the bagel's glycemic index because fat slows the impact of the bagel's carbohydrates on blood glucose. The degree to which a food is processed has an effect on its glycemic index, too. The smaller a food's particles are, the higher its glycemic index is. The glycemic index of a food is likely to rise the more it is processed, even in your own kitchen. For example, the glycemic index of instant rice nearly triples if you cook it for six minutes. In contrast, the more fiber a food contains, the lower its glycemic index; the index for brown rice, which still has its outer fibrous coating, is far lower than that of white rice.

The glycemic index is not a substitute if you are insulin resistant and know you should be counting your carbohydrate intake. But in a pinch, when you simply must eat and are presented with a range of less-than-optimal choices, selecting the foods with the lowest glycemic index is a wise course.

Micronutrients

Contained within the macronutrients are the micronutrients—vitamins, minerals, amino acids, and fatty acids (discussed in the section below entitled Using Fat for Energy) that determine how well our bodies work. This section provides a brief overview of the importance of some micronutrients. You will find references to books that will tell you more in Appendix C.

Vitamins are essential to our health and vigor. With the exception of vitamin D, which we obtain from exposure to sunlight, our bodies do not manufacture them; we get them from the food we eat. We don't usually think about vitamins unless we develop a deficiency in one. A vitamin deficiency can cause unpleasant symptoms, and it may even make us sick. People often take a daily multivitamin pill as insurance against deficiencies. That's not a bad idea, but it's a good bet that most general-purpose multivitamin preparations are formulated for some mythical average person, probably a healthy and active man in his thirties. We are each unique in our nutritional needs. A multivitamin may be better for you than nothing, but more effective is becoming familiar with the characteristics of deficiency in each vitamin to determine which, if any, you need to supplement. Your physician can order blood tests to measure the levels of all micronutrients in your body and help you decide the best way to overcome any deficiencies. The full complement of tests is expensive and unlikely to be covered by health insurance, but tracking down and correcting deficiencies yields excellent benefits. Although micronutrient supplementation can have an effect as potent as medicine, nutritional supplements are actually foods, not drugs.

It doesn't take much to develop a vitamin deficiency. For example, people in northern climates can develop a vitamin D deficiency in winter, especially if they don't drink milk, which is fortified with vitamin D by law. People who consume refined carbohydrates—primarily white sugar, white flour, and alcohol—can develop deficiencies in some B vitamins. The process that refines sugar and flour strips away the B vitamins that are required by the body to metabolize the remaining product. Refined carbohydrates therefore steal B vitamins from your tissues and cause deficiency. If you use tobacco, each cigarette you smoke steals about 75 milligrams of vitamin C. Fresh fruits and vegetables are rich sources of many vitamins, but shipping and storage practices can deplete those vitamins and render the fruits and vegetables little more than good-tasting fiber.

You would have to consume a huge number of vitamin pills and spend a great deal of money to overdose on B-complex vitamins and C, the water-soluble vitamins. These vitamins dissolve in water and wash out of your body in your urine if you take more than you need; they are not stored in your tissues. The main drawback to the shotgun approach to taking B vitamins and C is that you may have expensive urine. The sole exception is vitamin B_{12}, which can be stored in the liver, but there is no recorded toxic dose of B_{12}. On the other hand, the oil-soluble vitamins— A, D, and E—are dissolved by fats. This is another reason (besides your cells' and hormones' need for cholesterol) why you should not try to eliminate fats from your diet. The oil-soluble vitamins are stored in your liver and body fat and it is possible to overdose on them. The descriptions that follow provide the function of the vitamin, the recommended intake form (whether from food or pill), and, where appropriate, the highest safe dose. Water-soluble vitamins are measured in milligrams (mg) or micrograms (mcg). One milligram is 1/1,000 of a gram (g); a microgram is 1/1,000 of a milligram. Fat-soluble vitamins are measured in international units (IU).

Specific Vitamins

Vitamin A strengthens the skin, vision, bones, nails, and hair, and helps with resistance to viral infections. The suggested daily dose is 4,000 IU to 5,000 IU. The maximum safe dose is 25,000 IU. Beta-carotene is an acceptable substitute for vitamin A. It is A's precursor—that is, your body turns beta-carotene into vitamin A, but only to the extent that you need that vitamin. Fifteen IU of beta-carotene yields 25,500 IU of vitamin A. Even if you were to take enough beta-carotene to turn your skin orange (the sign of a toxic vitamin A overdose), you would not actually become toxic. Beta-carotene not used to make A has other uses in the body: combined with vitamins C and E it is a powerful antioxidant.

Vitamin B_1 (thiamine) helps convert carbohydrates into energy. It serves as a mild diuretic and helps the body deal with stress. The recommended dose is 100 mcg per day. B_2 (riboflavin) converts proteins and fats into energy and helps maintain healthy tissues. It also helps the body deal with stress. The suggested dose is 50 mg. B_3 (niacin) also promotes fat and protein metabolism, helps with stress, and promotes cardiovascular health. The suggested dose is 50 mg. Some people find that niacin causes facial flushing when taken in large doses. An alternative is niacinamide, which does not have this effect, but niacinamide does not have the same cardiovascular benefits. The facial flushing rarely lasts for more than an hour and usually stops after a week or so. B_5 (pantothenic acid) supports metabolism of other nutrients, especially amino acids, and participates in the synthesis of many hormones. It is also associated with nerve health. A daily dose of 200 mg is suggested. B_6 (pyridoxine) strengthens the immune system and plays a role in the transmission of nerve impulses. A deficiency can cause depression and the nerve pain often associated with carpal tunnel syndrome. The suggested daily dose is 150 mg. Several years ago newspapers reported a case of an overdose of B_6 that resulted in slurred speech and a stumbling gait. The man affected had been taking 6 g (6,000 mg) a day for several months. The symptoms disappeared once he stopped consuming such a huge dose. Vitamin B_{12} promotes nervous system health and the production of hemoglobin (the oxygen-carrying cells) in the blood. It is sometimes used to treat memory loss, depression, and insomnia. The suggested dose is 100 mcg per day. Folate (folic acid) also helps form hemoglobin; the suggested dose is 400 mcg. Biotin acts in metabolizing other nutrients in food and helps maintain healthy skin. The suggested dose is 50 mcg. Inositol, with a suggested dose of 50 mcg, reduces LDL ("bad") cholesterol, aids sleep, and helps reduce anxiety.

Vitamin C (ascorbic acid) fortifies the immune system, helps reduce the effects of physical and psychological stress, and may help reduce elevated cholesterol. Two grams (2,000 mg) is a suggested daily dose. More than 10 g (10,000 mg) may cause an upset stomach, diarrhea, and excess acidity in the bloodstream.

Vitamin D promotes the health of bones and teeth. It regulates the level of calcium in the blood and aids in the absorption and distribution of digested calcium. The suggested dose is 200 IU, with more during the dark winter months. There is evidence of a relationship between a deficiency in vitamin D and seasonal affective disorder (SAD), a form of depression. The maximum safe dose is 1,000 IU.

Vitamin E promotes health of the blood and aids circulation. The suggested daily dose is 400 IU. People with an exaggerated tendency to form blood clots may need extra vitamin E. The safe maximum is 1,200 IU.

If you choose to experiment with vitamins, you should first read more about them (you'll find a suggested reference in Appendix C). Then find your own optimal level by starting at the suggested dose and working up gradually toward the maximum, if you feel the need. You will discover what's best for you by paying attention to (and perhaps keeping notes on) how you feel each day. It may take between a few weeks and a few months to see the results you are looking for, so be patient and attentive.

Minerals

In 1985, *The New York Times* published the results of a chemical analysis of the human body for its mineral content. The value of these minerals, not counting the cost of extracting them, was set at about eight dollars. Calcium was listed as the most prevalent mineral, followed by potassium, phosphorus, sodium, sulfur, magnesium, and traces of several others. Mineral deficiencies are not nearly as common as vitamin deficiencies, partly because faulty storage and handling of foods is not as likely to destroy their mineral content. Vitamins and minerals often work together, so a deficiency in one may be related to a deficiency in the other. This section discusses some important minerals and what foods provide them.

Food is not the only source of dietary minerals. Unless you are drinking distilled or rain water, you are likely to obtain some minerals from your drinking water and the water you use in cooking. Aquifers—underground sources of water that feed wells and reservoirs—are usually pockets within rock formations. Water stored within rock leaches minerals from the rock and provides you with minerals. Hard water is rich in calcium and magnesium. If chlorine bleach in your laundry water leaves brown stains on fabrics, your water is high in iron.

Calcium is the most prevalent mineral in your body, with 3 to 5 pounds found in teeth and bones. About 20 percent of your bone calcium breaks down and is replaced each year. Estrogen is involved in the replacement of calcium. As we age, calcium replacement becomes less efficient, and the risk of osteopenia (bone loss) and osteoporosis (brittle bone disease) increases. Vitamins A, C, and D are essential to the absorption of dietary calcium. In addition to building strong bones and teeth, calcium helps regulate your heartbeat and aids in signal transmission among nerves. The best natural sources of calcium are dairy products, soybeans, sardines, salmon, kale, broccoli, collards, peanuts, walnuts, and sunflower seeds. Calcium is often combined with magnesium as a supplement in a ratio of two parts of calcium to one part of magnesium. As a supplement, calcium tends to be constipating while magnesium has laxative qualities.

Magnesium is necessary for the metabolism of vitamin C and calcium. It is important for converting blood sugar into energy and for the function of nerves and muscles. Magnesium helps the body handle stress and can aid in fighting depression. It is found in nuts, seeds, figs, dark green vegetables, and bananas.

Iron is necessary to metabolize B vitamins. It is also essential for the production of hemoglobin and certain enzymes. Deficiencies in iron and calcium are common among American women. Fatigue is one of the symptoms of iron-deficiency anemia. Iron is plentiful in organ meats and other red meat, egg yolks, nuts, beans, asparagus, and molasses. People who consume large quantities of coffee or tea risk interfering with iron absorption.

Phosphorus is present in every cell in the body. It requires vitamin D and calcium to function properly. Niacin cannot be absorbed without phosphorus, which is involved in virtually every chemical process within the body. It is important for kidney function, the transmission of nerve impulses, and regular heartbeat. Fortunately, phosphorus is easy to obtain from food sources: it is present in meat, fish, poultry, eggs, nuts, and seeds. The ideal balance between calcium and phosphorus is similar to that of calcium and magnesium: two parts of calcium to one of phosphorus. Soft drinks are high in phosphorus; overconsumption may lead to calcium depletion in your bones.

Potassium and sodium work together to regulate the body's water balance and heartbeat. The balance between potassium and sodium is crucial to the function of nerves and muscles. People who take thiazide diuretics are prone to potassium deficiency, which can manifest itself in irregular heartbeat. Potassium helps transport oxygen to the brain and aids in clear mental processing. It counteracts sodium's tendency to raise blood pressure. Food sources include citrus fruits, bananas, all green leafy vegetables, tomatoes, and cantaloupe.

A deficiency in sodium is rare because of the amount of table salt in the typical American diet. More common is a high intake of sodium, which depletes potassium. Sodium helps keep calcium and other minerals available in the bloodstream. Foods high in sodium include shellfish, carrots, beets, and cured meats such as ham and bacon. People who have high blood pressure should become aware of the sodium content of everything they eat. However, if you live in a hot climate and tend to sweat a lot, you should know that a sodium deficiency can lead to dehydration and heat prostration.

Zinc is essential for the synthesis of proteins, the maintenance of enzyme systems, and the production of new cells. It helps in the formation of insulin and is important in brain function. There is evidence that it is required in the synthesis of DNA and essential in DNA repair. Zinc aids in healing and helps minimize or avoid prostate problems. It is found in meat, organ meats, seafood, pumpkin seeds, and eggs.

Amino Acids

Amino acids are the building blocks of protein. As such, they are necessary to sustain life. A deficiency in one amino acid will reduce the effectiveness of all the others. Amino acids are the products of protein digestion. They combine with nitrogen to form thousands of different proteins in the body, from muscle tissue to hormones. There are twenty-two known amino acids, eight of which must be obtained from food or supplements because they cannot be manufactured by the human body. These eight, called the essential amino acids, are isoleucine, leucine, lysine, methionine, phenylalanine, threonine, tryptophan, and valine.

All protein foods are composed of amino acids, but foods differ in the way the various amino acids are represented. To form new proteins in the body, amino acids seek each other out and form chains. A protein is synthesized when a complete set of amino acids required for a particular protein is assembled with the essential and nonessential amino acids represented in the proper proportion. Amino acids that are present but not needed at the time join other chains or are carried off as waste. Some amino acids have properties that make them valuable for other purposes in addition to building new proteins. To obtain these benefits, the specific amino acids must be taken as nutritional supplements apart from a meal, so they don't link up with other amino acids to form a chain.

For example, the amino acids ornithine, arginine, tryptophan, glycine, and tyrosine work synergistically—that is, they are more effective together than individually—to stimulate the release of growth hormone during the night. To do this they require the presence of vitamin B_6, niacin, zinc, calcium, magnesium, potassium, and vitamin C. Ornithine and arginine are particularly effective as growth-hormone stimulators. In addition, ornithine stimulates insulin secretion and facilitates insulin's effect in building muscle. There is no need to take both ornithine and arginine because each triggers the synthesis of the other. In fact arginine is probably best obtained by taking ornithine.

A special caution is necessary with arginine, however: it is associated with oubreaks of the herpes virus. People who are subject to cold sores or genital herpes must be extra careful if they take either ornithine or arginine. Anyone who has had chicken pox, a form of the herpes virus, is susceptible to developing shingles later in life. The chicken pox virus lurks along the spinal nerves awaiting the opportunity afforded by a weakened immune system to break out as shingles. Arginine can trigger an attack of shingles in someone whose immune system has been weakened by illness or excessive stress. As a precaution, if you suspect you may be vulnerable to the herpes virus, you should add the amino acid lysine—an essential amino acid your body cannot synthesize on its own—to your amino acid regimen. Lysine is hostile to herpes and helps keep it under control. In men, seminal fluid contains up to 80 percent arginine, and this amino acid is thought to increase the sperm count.

Two other amino acids worth noting here are phenylalanine and DL-phenylalanine (DLPA). The two are related, but their functions are quite different. Phenylalanine is an essential amino acid that is the precursor to the nonessential amino acid tyrosine and also gives rise to the brain chemical dopamine. Tyrosine stimulates the thyroid to release its hormones and is associated with production of the adrenal hormone norepinephrine. Dopamine is a stimulating neurohormone linked to the brain's pleasure center. Dopamine also has much to do with the reduction of water retention. People low in dopamine and thyroid hormones do not perspire; taking phenylalanine as a nutritional supplement may promote sweating. A deficiency in dopamine is responsible for tremors and restless leg syndrome (in which the legs cannot keep still, disturbing rest and sleep). Tremors often associated with aging can be decreased with a daily dose of 500 to 1,000 mg of phenylalanine. Parkinson's disease is the result of a total failure of dopamine production. Research has yet to be done to determine whether treating Parkinson's patients with phenylalanine can cure or even retard the disease's progression.

The DL-phenylalanine molecule is actually a combination of the phenylalanine molecule and its mirror image. DLPA acts to prolong the action of endorphins in the brain. "Endorphin" is a shortening of the term "endogenous morphine." DLPA's molecular structure and shape are identical to morphine's, so that DLPA fits into the same receptors and acts to relieve chronic pain in the same way as the opioid drug. As is true with all body chemicals, an enzyme exists whose function is to break down endorphins. Without that enzyme, the brain would be overwhelmed with endorphins, and the result would be similar to morphine toxicity. DLPA inhibits the action of the enzyme that breaks down endorphins. It doesn't stop it from acting; it just makes it work more slowly. The result is naturally occurring relief from pain.

Because exercise increases the production of endorphins, people who exercise regularly get more benefit from DLPA than those who do not. The usual dose is 500 mg three times a day on an empty stomach. It is not a fast-acting pain reliever. Some people experience relief within twenty-four hours; others can take as long as three weeks. In cases of severe pain it may be necessary for you to continue whatever analgesia has been prescribed, tapering off gradually to determine whether DLPA is working. If relief is not attained within three weeks you can double the dose for another two to three weeks. If it still doesn't help, you are among the unfortunate 15 percent of people for whom DLPA provides no relief.

To get the best effect from amino acids taken for specific purposes, take them with water on an empty stomach—a half hour before or two hours after a meal. This prevents the amino acids from joining with others to form proteins. Tryptophan, another amino acid with specific properties, is discussed in the following section, which deals with the relationship between food and mood.

Diet and Mind

Just as the food you eat determines the composition of your body, it also has a profound influence on your mind. There is a direct connection between food and mood. For example, the habit of eating a diet loaded with carbohydrates often leads to insulin resistance, with its accompanying roller-coaster effect on blood sugar. If you tend to get cranky when you're hungry, that's because your blood sugar is low. People who learn to keep their blood sugar on an even keel don't get angry because it's time to eat. This peaks-and-valleys glucose mode can produce mild to moderate depression, which may lift during high-blood-sugar periods but come back with a vengeance when your glucose dips. You're apt to notice the valleys more than the peaks and think of yourself as chronically depressed, when the problem is really faulty diet.

Paradoxically, depression is the most common cause of overeating. The brain chemical most closely associated with both mood and appetite is serotonin, which is a product of the amino acid tryptophan. Tryptophan is also related to sleep and, in the circular way in which our body's chemistry so often acts, to the perception of pain. Each of these phenomena is worth exploring.

Foods rich in sugars and starches, especially those with a high glycemic index, deliver tryptophan faster than its more slowly metabolized meat sources. Tryptophan metabolizes into 5-hydroxytryptophan (5-HTP; more about that shortly) and then into serotonin. In this way, fast-acting carbohydrates raise serotonin levels quickly. A high serotonin level makes people feel good. Therefore, many people eat to feel better, not because they are hungry. Serotonin surges result in a conditioned response, and in some cases, compulsive overeating. Carbohydrates can become a kind of drug that causes people to engage in binge eating out of an unconscious desire to increase the level of serotonin in the brain.

A low level of serotonin in the brain is closely associated with depression. Here's another one of those cyclical phenomena: Something—perhaps stress, perhaps a leaky gut that prevents you from absorbing nutrients efficiently—lowers your serotonin level. You eat more, mostly carbohydrates, to alleviate your depression by raising your serotonin. Your eating habits make you gain weight. The weight gain, coupled with your apparent inability to control your eating, increases your stress. The resulting stress hormones deplete serotonin, so you become more depressed, which further lowers your serotonin level, and the cycle continues. We'll discuss a way to break this cycle shortly.

When serotonin is low, sleep is apt to be unsatisfactory. Serotonin helps you relax into sleep. Deep, restorative sleep is necessary to undo the stresses of the day. Poor sleep elevates pain by triggering the release of excess cytokines, the immune system cells implicated in muscle aches. Insomnia also interferes with the release of growth hormone; growth hormone, which relieves some muscle pain, also brings about the anti-aging benefits already discussed. Improving sleep is an important component of any age-management program.

The perception of pain in the brain is handled by a chemical known as substance P. There is an inverse relationship between serotonin and substance P. Therefore, when serotonin is plentiful, the perception of pain decreases. To be sure, the ability to perceive pain is necessary to maintain health and life itself. Pain warns us of injury and infection so we can take steps to repair ourselves. But the heightened perception of pain brought about by low serotonin and high substance P is far from helpful. In addition to being distressing in itself and leading to depression, people who frequently complain of pain that has no discernable cause risk alienating those around them, including their physicians. The same technique that can break the cycle of depression and overeating can lower the exaggerated perception of pain brought about by excessive substance P.

The nutritional approach to these three interrelated problems is to increase the production of serotonin in the brain. Before 1990, many people did this by taking the amino acid tryptophan, which breaks down into 5-HTP and then into serotonin. (A small portion of serotonin resolves into melatonin, the body clock hormone.) Then an outbreak of tryptophan-related illness and several deaths occurred in the United States. The U.S. Food and Drug Administration (FDA) ordered the amino acid off the market until the source of the illness was identified. However, the FDA refused to allow sale of the amino acid to resume once the cause was discovered to be contamination in a single Japanese company's manufacturing process. Today tryptophan is available for use only in infant formulas, in nutritional mixtures fed through a stomach tube, and in animal feeds. Healthy people cannot buy it without a doctor's prescription, a trip to Canada, or without lying about its purpose.

5-HTP, the breakdown product of tryptophan, is readily available without a prescription in drugstores and natural food stores, both the brick-

and-mortar variety and those on the Internet. People use it, usually with success, to relieve mild-to-moderate depression, improve their sleep, reduce pain, and control a runaway appetite for carbohydrates. 5-HTP does not need to be taken on an empty stomach, unlike tryptophan and other amino acids. Doses range from 50 mg to 600 mg, depending on the purpose, the severity of the problem, and probably one's genetic makeup. The ratio of tryptophan to 5-HTP is 3 to 1, so people who took 1,500 mg of L-tryptophan before it was banned will probably do well with 300 mg of 5-HTP. The best course is to start with 50 mg to 100 mg and work up gradually until you achieve the result you're looking for. One of the most beneficial results of improving your serotonin level is that it becomes easier to give up a high-carbohydrate diet. Once you do that, your cravings and overeating will come to an end.

USING FAT FOR ENERGY

If you adopt a low-carbohydrate nutrition plan, as this book recommends, and you find you need to consume fewer than about 90 grams of carbohydrate to combat insulin resistance, you are likely to enter a physical state in which most of your energy is derived from burning fat rather than glucose. This state is known as *ketosis;* it is the subject of considerable controversy and even more misinformation. This section explains the facts about ketosis and strips away the myths surrounding it.

Your body can derive energy from all the macronutrients. Carbohydrates provide the quickest energy boost because they are converted into glucose almost immediately. Glucose is stored in the liver and muscle cells as glycogen for future use. (If you are insulin resistant, surplus glucose will also be stored as fat, because glycation prevents glucose molecules from connecting with the receptors meant to conduct them into muscle cells.) Protein's main purpose is to replenish the body's tissues. It can also be converted into glucose in the liver through a process known as *gluconeogenesis* (*neo* means "new," and *genesis* means "creation," so *gluconeogenesis* means "making new glucose"). Fat is stored as triglycerides, mainly in body fat, where it can be broken down into glycerol and free fatty acids (FFAs) to be burned for energy. When fat cells are full, excess fat shows up as triglycerides in the bloodstream. Your nutritional state and your metab-

Diabetes and Ketosis

Type 1 diabetes is a disease in which the pancreas does not produce insulin on its own. People with this condition must inject themselves with insulin several times a day. Since their bodies have no mechanism for regulating blood sugar, injected insulin is their only choice. For Type 1 diabetics, ketosis can indeed be dangerous. The proper term for the condition in which a Type 1 diabetic burns fat instead of glucose is *diabetic ketoacidosis*. That's where some confusion may arise. Equating diabetic ketoacidosis with ketosis is simply inaccurate since the processes by which the two work are entirely different. Diabetic ketoacidosis is a life-threatening situation that happens only to people with Type 1 diabetes. Dietary ketosis is not dangerous; in fact, it is more likely to be life enhancing.

Many people, including Type 2 diabetics, have discovered that the state of ketosis is the best way for them to control their blood sugar. Even Type 2 diabetics who use insulin may be able to wean themselves off injections with care. As long as you have a working pancreas, you may want to discuss a low-carbohydrate diet and the possible advantages of dietary ketosis with your physician.

Here's the difference between ketosis and diabetic ketoacidosis: Nondiabetics and Type 2 diabetics go into dietary ketosis when blood glucose is low. Diabetics go into ketoacidosis when blood glucose is too high, usually because they have been without insulin for too long, or have used it up too quickly by exercising with unaccustomed vigor. When ketones accumulate in amounts that threaten to make the blood dangerously acidic, a functioning pancreas responds with a surge of glucagon, the fat-burning hormone, which lowers blood ketones to a safe level. The pancreas of a Type 1 diabetic cannot counteract ketosis before it becomes dangerous ketoacidosis. The ketone strips that low-carbohydrate dieters use to monitor their ketone levels (see "Measuring Ketones" on page 99) are actually intended for Type 1 diabetics to use to ensure that they are not heading toward ketoacidosis.

olism determine the proportion in which these forms of energy are used. If carbohydrates predominate in your diet, insulin will see to it that glucose is your primary energy source. If carbohydrates are scarce, the insulin/glucagon balance tips in favor of glucagon. Glucagon's preferred energy source is FFAs.

To say that your body will burn glucose first if it is available is not the same as saying your body prefers to burn glucose; it's just easier. Except for a portion of your brain, a part of your eyes, and a piece of your kidneys, your body has no preference. When glucose stores run low, your liver breaks down FFAs, producing a byproduct known as ketone bodies, or ketones. Your brain cannot use FFAs, but it is perfectly happy to use ketones in addition to whatever glucose happens to be available. Some experts say that ketones exist to provide energy to the brain when glucose is scarce. In fact, researchers have discovered that your brain runs with 25 percent greater efficiency when it burns fat for energy. Some ketones are always present in a person who does not have diabetes, and in a Type 2 diabetic with well-controlled blood sugar. A high-carbohydrate intake, however, keeps the concentration of ketones too low to measure.

Your body uses up its store of glucose in about twenty-four hours when you eat little or no carbohydrate-containing foods. Then your liver turns on the gluconeogenesis process, using protein to produce the glucose your brain needs. If your diet contains sufficient protein, your liver will use some of it to produce glucose; if you are fasting, your liver will start drawing protein from your muscles to create glucose. Within another twenty-four hours or so it will start looking for fat to burn, producing FFAs and ketones. When this state of ketosis is reached, ketones show up in the bloodstream and in the urine.

Ketosis may be nature's answer to the thrifty gene theory. Our hunter-gatherer ancestors were probably in ketosis most of the time, since they had few carbohydrates available until they adopted agriculture and began growing grains. Until we started eating cereal grains and starches, Type 2 diabetes was unknown, and those born with Type 1 diabetes and a non-functioning pancreas didn't live very long.

The term for a diet so low in carbohydrate that it puts you into ketosis is a *ketogenic diet*. Children who suffer from epileptic seizures that cannot be controlled with medication are often put on a ketogenic diet, in which they are fed nothing but fat. How this works is not well understood, but there seems to be some relationship between glucose and the irritation of the brain that results in epileptic seizures. The main argument against the ketogenic diet for epileptics is that it is difficult to sustain, and preparing meals requires considerable work and careful measurement. No one claims that the diet is dangerous for epileptic children. It is difficult to understand why some doctors tell their adult patients that a ketogenic diet will ruin their kidneys or cause clogged arteries. Actually, the opposite is the case. People who follow a low-carbohydrate regimen, especially one providing glucose levels low enough to cause ketosis, usually find that their blood pressure goes down, their triglyceride and low-density ("bad") lipoprotein levels decrease, and their overall cholesterol count improves. It is carbohydrates, not dietary fats, that cause high cholesterol and all the associated risks.

Ketosis will not hurt your kidneys, although people with end-stage kidney disease must not eat a diet high in protein, which is the corollary

Measuring Ketones

It is possible and may be desirable to measure the ketone content of your urine while you adjust your carbohydrate intake. To do this you can purchase ketone test strips at any drugstore. The end of each strip contains a chemical that changes color when it is dipped into a urine specimen or held in the urine stream. The darker the color—the range is from light pink to purple—the higher the concentration of ketones. A color scale on the container of strips helps you interpret the results. Dark purple does not mean you are doing better or losing weight faster. It simply means you have more ketones in your urine, possibly because you are eating more fat than you need for energy. It is best to keep the color in the moderate range if part of your goal of being in ketosis is to lose weight and redistribute your fat in more esthetically pleasing ways. Of course, if your bloodstream doesn't carry a heavy load of glucose, glycation ceases to be a problem.

of a low-carbohydrate diet. If your kidneys are reasonably healthy, you need take only one precaution: to prevent kidney stones, you should drink at least eight 8-ounce glasses of water each day. It is said you can spot the people on low-carbohydrate diets on the subway; they're the ones carrying bottles of water.

Caloric Restriction

It bears repeating that a low-carbohydrate diet is not the same as a weight-loss diet. Still, if you are overweight, you will almost certainly lose weight if you replace a significant portion of your customary carbohydrate intake with proteins. Gram for gram, proteins and carbohydrates are identical in terms of the number of calories (energy) they provide. But the body's glucose and insulin response to proteins is drastically different from its response to carbohydrates. The difference explains why reducing carbohydrates reduces body weight.

Another anti-aging stratagem that dramatically reduces body weight is attracting increasing attention. Caloric restriction with adequate nutrition (CRAN, or simply CR) involves reducing your caloric intake by as much as 30 percent, while being sure to provide your body with all the vitamins and other nutrients essential to support life. What this means is that an adult who takes in 2,500 calories a day would cut back to a daily intake of 1,750 calories. This is almost twice the 900 calories most adult bodies require to carry out the basic processes of life: digestion, metabolism, blood and lymph circulation, respiration, and the like. But few people can sustain the discipline required to cut their food intake by nearly one-third all at once. To do so and then revert to the higher-calorie level is not much different from yo-yo dieting that causes increased weight gain and the other ill effects previously discussed. A more realistic approach to CR is to cut your intake by 10 percent, adapt to that, and then cut another 10 percent. After you've adjusted again, do it once more. This more gradual approach is less likely to disturb your body's homeostasis—its wish to keep everything on an even keel—and trigger the emergency response system that elevates stress hormones and slows metabolism to conserve energy.

Although CR has yet to undergo scientific testing in human beings, there is convincing evidence from studies of other living beings to suggest that CR offers numerous anti-aging advantages. Laboratory tests on single-celled animals, guppies, spiders, and rodents have demonstrated that cutting their caloric intake while still providing the nutrients they need extends their lives significantly. In one experiment, giving lab rats about two-thirds of the calories they would eat if they had unrestricted access to food extended their average life span by 30 percent. Not only did the animals live longer, but they also showed signs of improved health: they learned to run mazes faster and had better biomarkers of aging, such as blood pressure, HDL cholesterol and triglyceride levels, and insulin and DHEA levels. Similar studies are currently underway using rhesus and squirrel monkeys, which are biologically closer to human beings than rats. Since these monkeys have a normal life span of twenty to thirty years, the results for primates won't be known for a long time, but early test indications strongly suggest the same positive results.

From what has been observed so far in the animals tested, caloric restriction seems to decrease much of the metabolic damage associated with aging, reducing glycation and oxidative harm. CR also appears to slow the ill effects of aging on the nervous system, reproductive organs, and the production of hormones. In addition, CR blunts the damaging effects of hyperthermia (overheating) in the mammals that have been tested. Mammals produce protective substances known as heat-shock proteins that prevent them from overheating. In older mammals, the ability to produce these proteins is reduced, which is why old people are more likely to die in a prolonged heat wave. CR has been shown to enhance the body's ability to synthesize heat-shock proteins. The negative side of CR is that calorie-restricted animals tend to have a reduced ability to deal with hypothermia (lowered body temperature), which is another environmental hazard to which human beings become more vulnerable as they age.

Although it is too early to state with certainty that CR is beneficial to human beings, two bits of anecdotal evidence suggest that this is the case. During the Biosphere 2 experiment in Arizona in 1993–1994, the eight participants found themselves unable to grow enough food to sustain a normal diet. Thus, they underwent an unintentional CR experiment for nearly two years. A member of the Biosphere 2 team conducted regular physiological and biochemical measurements of the crew members and found anti-aging biomarkers similar to those already found in rodents and monkeys that had been tested. In addition, the inhabitants of the Japanese island of Okinawa traditionally consume a diet 20 percent lower in calories on average than people in mainland Japan. A study done in the 1970s found that death rates from stroke were 41 percent lower on the island than on the mainland, cancer deaths were 31 percent lower, and heart attack deaths 41 percent lower. Half as many people between the ages of sixty and sixty-four died on the island as on the mainland, and the number of people living to the age of 100 or more was reported to be forty times greater than in the rest of Japan.

If your body composition is already ideal, cutting your caloric intake is not a good idea. Nor is CR for you if you despair of having the discipline to maintain a CR regimen for the rest of your life, or if you show evidence of having the thrifty gene. Fortunately, science suggests an alternative— the anti-diabetic drug metformin (its brand name is Glucophage). In one study, metformin and three other blood-sugar-regulating drugs were fed to elderly mice while other groups of mice were subjected to short- and long-term CR, and a fourth group was kept as a control (allowed to feed normally and given no medicinal drugs). The results showed that both use of metformin and CR resulted in altered gene expression linked to improved energy metabolism, protein synthesis, and cell growth and replacement. Another study concluded that metformin extended the life span of mice by 20 percent. Also, a recent study demonstrates that metformin combats inflammation. These findings suggest that metformin does more than regulate blood sugar and insulin; it may be a real anti-aging drug.

No human studies have been performed to determine the optimal dose of metformin for any anti-aging purpose. People may differ genetically in their response to the drug. Blood tests should be performed at the start of metformin therapy, and periodically while it continues. The tests include a fasting insulin, to determine the baseline level of insulin in your blood; a CBC (complete blood count/blood chemistry panel that includes fasting glucose, triglycerides, and liver- and kidney-function indicators); and a test of hemoglobin A1c, which measures the average amount of glucose in your blood over the previous six weeks to three months.

EXERCISE AND AGING

Like proper nutrition, exercise is essential to controlling hormone levels that combat premature aging. Exercise is also one of the primary means of controlling body composition—the ratio of lean muscle to fat—as well as bringing about positive changes in quality of life and improving all levels of functioning. Most of the key biomarkers of aging are improved with exercise; even those that do not increase longevity improve our lives in many ways. Exercise builds muscle and muscle burns more calories than fat. Increasing the rate at which glucose is burned reduces glycation and makes cells more receptive to insulin. Contrary to what many people think, exercise provides more energy, not less, because it counters insulin resistance and makes the mitochondria in the cells more efficient at energy production. Lowered glucose in the blood also reduces the need for insulin and elevates the ratio of glucagon—the fat-burning hormone—to insulin. This hormonal change sets off a cascade of biochemical events that have beneficial effects on the aging equation and the quality and repair of our DNA. Among the most important hormone effects are elevations of growth-hormone secretion and testosterone in both men and women. Exercise also improves cardiovascular function, strengthens

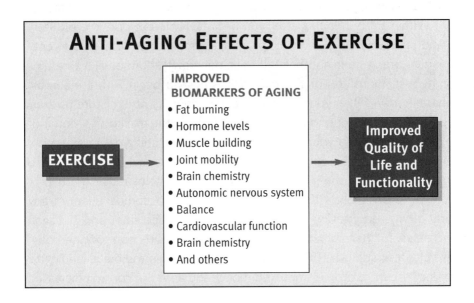

ANTI-AGING EFFECTS OF EXERCISE

EXERCISE →

IMPROVED BIOMARKERS OF AGING
• Fat burning
• Hormone levels
• Muscle building
• Joint mobility
• Brain chemistry
• Autonomic nervous system
• Balance
• Cardiovascular function
• Brain chemistry
• And others

→ **Improved Quality of Life and Functionality**

bones, improves cognitive function, and leads to improved coordination and sense of balance.

There are four categories of exercise, two major and two minor. The major categories are aerobic and anaerobic exercise. The minor ones are stretching and breathing. This section discusses all four forms of exercise and why each is important.

Aerobic Exercise

Aerobic exercise is the sort that makes our hearts beat faster and our rate of breathing increase. Walking is a form of aerobic exercise. Recent studies have shown that fat loss can result simply from a long-term walking program without any dieting. Vigorous walking reduces stores of body fat and insulin demand in both animal and human experiments. Other forms of aerobic exercise include jogging; running; bicycling, whether on a moving or stationary bike; walking on a treadmill; using a stair-climber or elliptical machine; and high- and low-impact aerobic dance. Breathing faster increases lung capacity and promotes endurance. After only a few weeks of an aerobic-exercise regimen you will find it easier to climb stairs without becoming winded. Aerobic exercise stimulates an increased demand for oxygen and results in the formation of additional capillaries surrounding the heart, giving you an extra measure of protection from a heart attack.

Within thirty minutes after you begin aerobic exercise, the pituitary gland releases a surge of HGH, peaking approximately fifteen to twenty minutes later. Within another half hour, the growth-hormone level returns to its baseline value. For this reason, it is best to begin with the aerobic phase on days when your exercise program consists of a mixture of exercise forms, as it should on most days. This brings the maximum amount of oxygen and heat to your muscles and makes stretching easier and more effective. Stretching cold muscles is far from optimal and can lead to injury. In addition, the surge of growth hormone helps repair the microscopic tears in muscle tissue that are the normal accompaniment of any kind of vigorous motion. As you exercise, insulin decreases and glucagon increases, further stimulating the release of growth hormone. Aerobic exercise also stimulates the release of endorphins in the brain, leading to an increase in serotonin, improved mood, and appetite control. Increased serotonin also improves the quality of your sleep, but only if your workout takes place no less than four hours before sleep. Closer to your sleep time, vigorous exercise is apt to be more stimulating than relaxing.

Your goal in terms of heart rate should be between 60 and 80 percent of your maximum heart rate. To calculate this, subtract your age from 220, then figure both 60 and 80 percent of the resulting number. For example, here is the formula if you are fifty:

$$220 - 50 = 170 \quad \bullet \quad 60\% \text{ of } 170 = 102 \quad \bullet \quad 80\% \text{ of } 170 = 136$$

Thus, your optimal heart rate during aerobic exercise should be between 102 and 136 beats per minute. You can check your heart rate while you exercise by finding your pulse, using the first two fingers of your right hand pressed lightly against your left wrist below the thumb joint. Count pulses for ten seconds and multiply by six to get the number of beats in a minute. Some exercise machines monitor your heart rate if you put both hands on their sensors.

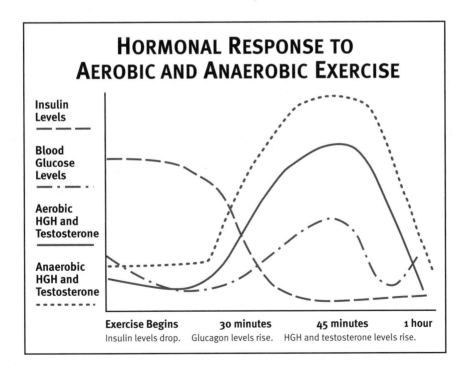

HORMONAL RESPONSE TO AEROBIC AND ANAEROBIC EXERCISE

Insulin Levels

Blood Glucose Levels

Aerobic HGH and Testosterone

Anaerobic HGH and Testosterone

Exercise Begins　　　**30 minutes**　　　**45 minutes**　　**1 hour**

Insulin levels drop.　Glucagon levels rise.　HGH and testosterone levels rise.

If you are new to aerobic exercise, you should check with your physician and see if you need to have a physical exam before starting. In any case, you should start slowly, and stop before breathing becomes difficult. During any exercise period your activity should never become so vigorous that you cannot carry on a conversation while you exercise. If you walk or run with a companion, it's easy to converse occasionally as a check on your safety and that of the other person. If you exercise alone, one way to be sure you're not getting too out of breath is to recite a nursery rhyme in a low tone of voice. This doesn't go over too well if you work out in a club—people may get the wrong idea about your mental status—but you may have a trainer to keep an eye on you there. Never exercise aerobically to the point where you become light-headed or feel nauseated. Find a level of exercise that is comfortable for you, and stay there until it becomes easy. Then increase your exercise by 10 to 20 percent (measured in time or repetitions, depending on the form of exercise) and stay at that level until it, too, feels easy. Ideally, your aerobic workout will eventually last between twenty and thirty minutes, at least five days a week.

Anaerobic Exercise

Anaerobic, or resistive, exercise includes weight lifting and calisthenics. In addition to stimulating release of growth hormone and testosterone, resistive exercise strengthens bone and reduces the likelihood of osteoporosis. Anaerobic exercise also improves muscle mass and the distribution of fat. Within minutes of beginning a session of weight lifting or calisthenics, a surge of growth hormone and testosterone occurs. The effects of this surge last for forty-five to sixty minutes. The resulting improvement in muscle tone and the strength of tendons and ligaments lasts for as long as you maintain your exercise regimen.

The ideal resistive exercise session will last no more than forty-five minutes, two or three times a week. There is no benefit, and there may even be a disadvantage, to an anaerobic exercise session lasting more than forty-five minutes. At that point, cortisol levels begin to increase to the extent that other hormone functions tend to become impaired. The increase in cortisol causes an increase in blood sugar, stimulating additional insulin production. At the same time, excessive exercise triggers a drop in production of DHEA and a resulting decrease in release of testosterone. Free-radical production may also be accelerated, with the negative effect that oxidative stress implies. These effects are detrimental to your anti-aging program.

Stretching and Breathing

Both stretching and breathing should be part of any age-management program. Do your stretching after your aerobic workout, and also on the days you do no other exercise. Deep breathing is not normally considered exercise, but it can be valuable in improving several reversible biomarkers of aging.

Stretching improves flexibility of the spine and the major joint complexes of the hip and shoulder girdle and keeps limbs and joints supple. It stimulates release of the synovial fluid that bathes the joints and keeps them lubricated. Stretching also stimulates increased flow of blood and lymph, improving circulation to the brain and other organs and strengthening the immune system. Certain yoga postures that have been popular for virtually thousands of years help to accomplish all these goals and improve blood flow to the digestive organs, particularly the liver and pancreas. The daily practice of stretching also helps keep the spinal column in alignment, which is essential to avoid nerve and disc injuries and low back pain so common in older people. On the days you don't work out, stretching should be part of your routine.

Slow, deliberate, deep breathing can, over time, improve pulmonary functions and oxygen delivery to the tissues while removing excess acidity and helping to balance pH of the blood and cellular fluids. Deep breathing—moving the abdomen, not the chest—also produces marked relaxation of the central nervous system (CNS), putting you in a calmer, more focused, mental state. Whether this breathing is performed in conjunction with yoga postures or on its own, the effects of a focused breathing session on many of the biomarkers of aging have been documented to be extremely beneficial. Deep breathing can be done at any time and can be a potent stress-reducing technique. Two of the best times to practice deep breathing are when you are in bed before falling asleep and when you are in your car, stuck in a traffic jam. Appendix C suggests books on stretching and breathing.

AGE-MANAGEMENT ESSENTIALS: DIET AND EXERCISE

Diet and exercise are the twin essentials of a successful age-management program. If your body composition—the ratio of lean muscle to fat—is not what you want it to be, reduce your intake of carbohydrates and increase your intake of proteins until you get to the point where you are losing weight at a satisfying rate (a pound or two a week, after the initial larger weight loss, which is mostly water released by your tissues). Pay attention to signs of vitamin and mineral deficiencies and take steps to correct any that develop or exist. Think about the benefits of amino acids both for body building and improvement in hormone levels. Eat the best quality, least processed foods you can. Avoid simple sugars like the plague.

Develop—gradually and gently, if you are a sedentary being—a program of stretching, aerobic and anaerobic exercise, and deep breathing. The results will be gratifying: reduction and redistribution of fat; improvement in muscle mass, strength, coordination, and endurance; improved joint mobility and spinal integrity; enhanced cardiovascular function; a better-balanced autonomic (involuntary) nervous system and improved brain chemistry; and overall improvement in the biomarkers of aging and the protection and repair of your DNA.

Age management is a matter of choice, regardless of your present age. It is never too late to start.

CHAPTER 7

Anti-Aging Treatments and Technologies

EVERYTHING SHOULD BE MADE AS SIMPLE AS POSSIBLE,
BUT NOT SIMPLER.
—*Albert Einstein*

The first human being to live to be 200 years old is walking the planet today. It may be one of our children, or perhaps even one of our own generation. Today's anti-aging regimen and associated treatments can prolong healthy life for almost anyone, regardless of age. Emerging technologies, some of which are available today, improve the promise of extending life beyond anything previous generations could have imagined.

The fundamental processes by which we age form a complex equation encoded in our twenty-three chromosome pairs. Breaking the aging code consists of minimizing glycation, inflammatory processes, and oxidative stress, while improving the process of methylation to regulate gene expression, minimize DNA damage, and maximize DNA repair. The lifestyle modifications set out in this book provide most of the building blocks required to achieve our longevity goals. If you want to go further, additional benefits are possible through pharmaceutical intervention, which requires the assistance of a skilled aging-management professional. (The American Academy of Anti-Aging Medicine, listed in Appendix B, can help you find an appropriate practitioner.) Taken together, the measures described here will have the most positive impact possible on the aging equation. They influence hormonal levels, restoring a more youthful balance and function to the endocrine, immune, digestive, and central nervous systems. In this way, the body's systems learn again what they knew when we were young—how to integrate with each other, providing the balance and homeostasis that sustains life at its best.

With the increased knowledge and understanding we have gained by breaking the aging code, we have at hand a new way of looking at aging. No matter how we have treated ourselves in the past, this new paradigm enables us to live longer, healthier, more productive lives. This chapter details the treatments and technologies that can help make that possible.

GENE EXPRESSION AND CELL SIGNALING

Research in the last several years has documented the success of using nutraceuticals—vitamins, minerals, amino acids, plant phytochemicals, and enzyme complexes—as well as prescription drugs, to directly influence gene expression. When done correctly, downregulating some genes and upregulating others can adjust the synthesis of enzymes that alter cell signaling and thus directly affect hormonal levels. Hormones are ultimately responsible for the changes in proteins and other growth factors that result in a favorable rate of tissue regeneration and other physical changes.

Glycation

Supplements that improve insulin sensitivity aid in controlling glycation. These include alpha-lipoic acid (ALA), vanadium, chromium, zinc, taurine, and the herbs fenugreek and bitter gourd. Metformin (Glucophage) is an efficient way to control the loss of insulin receptor sensitivity and resulting elevation of blood sugar levels. It also replaces the more onerous practice of calorie restriction by mimicking the effects of a reduced calorie diet. For this purpose the usual prescription is 125 mg two times a day, with lunch and dinner, which is less than 10 percent of the maximum dose prescribed for Type 2 diabetics. Aminoguanidine (brand name Wytensin), a drug normally used to lower blood pressure, is another medication that can help inhibit glycation and also support the immune system. The recommended amount is 200 mg twice daily, which is half the usual starting dose of 400 mg twice daily when it is used to treat high blood pressure.

Neither of these drugs nor any other compound mentioned in this chapter eliminates the need for a lifestyle that inhibits glycation—an optimal balance of low-glycemic-index carbohydrates, proteins, and fats, and a program of regular exercise.

Antioxidants

An antioxidant program is essential to help control DNA-damaging free-radical production, which is an unavoidable part of energy metabolism. Antioxidant supplements containing vitamins A, C, E, selenium, and zinc, and natural compounds from vegetable-derived foods are essential. The rate and quantity of DNA damage are directly related to elevated free-radical levels at both the nuclear and the cell-membrane levels. Experimental studies have shown that selegiline hydrochloride (brand name Deprenyl), an anti-tremor drug most commonly used to treat Parkinson's disease, improves levels of the intrinsic antioxidant compounds that we normally produce on our own. The suggested dosage for antioxidant support is 2.5 to 5.0 mg/day, which is one-quarter to one-half the standard dose. Other antioxidant compounds such as superoxide dismutase (SOD), catalase, and glutathione peroxidase are produced within the cells and the mitochondria, which is where most free-radical production and free-radical damage takes place.

Inflammation

Controlling the inflammatory process centers around a diet free of foods to which you are allergic, supplemented with digestive enzymes. These enzymes break down proteins into amino acids and aid in their absorption. If you suffer from frequent bouts of indigestion, you would do well to eliminate suspect foods for several weeks. Introduce them back into your diet one at a time, waiting for two or three weeks between introductions to see if allergic symptoms recur. The two classes of foods most likely to cause allergic reactions in adults are those containing wheat and dairy products. Many people have achieved relief from acid indigestion (gastric esophageal reflux disorder, or GERD) by eliminating wheat and dairy from their diets. It is important to know that most cases of indigestion in people of middle age and older result from overconsumption of carbohydrates, accompanied by insufficient digestive enzymes, not from lack of stomach acids. Although we are bombarded by advertisements telling us we have excess gastric juices that need to be controlled, this is simply not true for most of us. Gastrointestinal support with digestive enzymes, friendly digestive bacteria (acidophilus, bifidus, and lactobacillus) and amino acids such as L-glutamine can markedly decrease inflammatory processes occurring at the cellular level.

Maintaining an appropriate ratio of omega-6 and omega-3 essential fatty acids is another important way to regulate the inflammatory pathways within cells. Niacin or niacinamide and folic acid are natural approaches. Lipoic acid, boswellic acid, turmeric, gymnema, ginger, borage oil, and bitter gourd also help minimize inflammatory tendencies. Decreasing the burden of toxic elements such as aluminum, copper, and iron, which are found in drinking water in some areas, as well as in foods cooked in pots made of these metals, helps reduce the presence of inflammation. Celecoxib (brand name Celebrex), a class of anti-inflammatory drug that inhibits the enzyme that produces inflammatory eicosanoids, is useful when taken in doses of 50 to 100 mg once or twice a day. This is a quarter to a half the amount recommended to treat osteoarthritis. A water-soluble extract of cat's claw (uña de gato) is a medicinal herb credited with inhibiting both NF-κB and tumor necrosis factor alpha (TNF-α), both of which promote inflammation and the growth of tumors.

Methylation

Turning genes on and off at appropriate times is the result of proper methylation. It is facilitated by supplementation with vitamins B_6, B_{12}, folic acid, and the digestive aids betaine and glycine. Lowering excessive cortisol levels also improves methylation. The easiest way to do that is by augmenting DHEA, which decreases body fat as well as age-related brain-cell death associated with memory impairment. Only take DHEA under an age-management practitioner's supervision.

Energy Production

Another essential approach to anti-aging treatment is to improve mitochondrial production of ATP, the essential energy intermediate from which all cellular processes, including DNA repair, are accomplished. Keeping ATP production optimal is paramount in the effort to decelerate aging. This can be accomplished with lipoic acid, N-acetylcysteine, niacinamide, co-enzyme Q_{10}, lipoic acid, L-carnitine, taurine, vitamin E, and glutathione.

Immunity

Improving immune function can be accomplished with natural components from yeast cell extracts known as beta-1,3-glucans. The herbal compounds echinacea, goldenseal, and astragalus have all been documented to improve T-cell and immune functions, but studies have shown that echinacea diminishes in effectiveness if taken daily over a long period of time. It is better to take this herb for two or three weeks and then put it aside for a week or two. Reishi mushroom extract and shiitake mushroom concentrate are well-known immune stimulants as well.

Other Improvements

The composition of our cells is made up of 98 percent water; water is the medium in which all biochemical processes take place. It is essential to have the appropriate quantity and quality of water for this reason. Eight 8-ounce glasses of water are recommended for proper hydration. If you wait to drink water until you are thirsty, you're already dehydrated. Healthful water should tend toward the alkaline, which helps balance pH levels both within and between cells. That poses a particular problem in areas where acid rain provides much of the local water supply. Limestone filters exist that can transform acidic water to a more beneficial pH. Water softeners improve water surface tension and wetting ability and enhance cell-membrane permeability and cell hydration, allowing cellular wastes to leave and essential nutrients and electrolytes to enter the cells. Filters that soften water and raise its pH can be attached to the main water intake or to individual faucets.

Improving digestive function is another step in a program to deter aging. Simple maneuvers such as chewing food well and avoiding excessive carbohydrate consumption can help ameliorate leaky gut syndrome, a common condition in old age. Chewing thoroughly aids digestion by giving the gastrointestinal tract smaller bits of food to deal with. Increasing the intake of high-fiber foods is also important. Fiber helps increase the movement of food through the digestive system and prevents the ill effects of having waste material stay in contact with the intestinal walls for longer than necessary to absorb nutrients. The interaction between intestinal wastes and the lining of the lower bowel has been implicated in some cases of bowel cancer. A healthy complement of intestinal flora (the digestive bacteria acidophilus, bifidus, and lactobacillus) is essential to good digestive health. It is important to remember that antibiotics kill beneficial bacteria while they fight bacterial infections, so if you must take an antibiotic, you should take a digestive bacteria preparation at the same time. Jerusalem artichoke (a starchy vegetable nothing like an artichoke) contains substances that provide a hospitable medium for the growth of helpful intestinal bacteria.

HORMONE-REPLACEMENT PROTOCOLS

Hormone-replacement therapy can be a valuable component of an age-management program. It can help regulate and maintain such vital functions as the maintenance of bone mass, healthy levels of blood fats, and protection from cardiovascular disease. No one should embark on a hormone replacement program, however, without first having the necessary laboratory tests and without the supervision and advice of a qualified healthcare professional.

There is no place in anti-aging therapy for single-hormone replacement. In fact, replacement of growth hormone or testosterone alone can be deleterious to the aging process and longevity. Estrogen replacement has been in the news lately, with discouraging reports. The body is designed to act in concert and balance with all hormones in appropriate ratios. Changes in the level of a single hormone can trigger a cascade of effects that upsets the delicate balance of the neuroendocrine system. Therefore, it is essential to view hormone levels as an interdependent web. A complete hormone assay should be undertaken before a program of adjusting hormone levels is started. There is no "one size fits all" solution to hormone imbalance. The discussion that follows assumes deficiency in the hormones named. The recommendations should not be assumed to be appropriate for any particular individual without the evidence of laboratory tests.

Growth Hormone

HGH replacement therapy is accomplished with the use of recombinant growth hormone, 0.5 to 1 unit per day. It is recommended that the hormone be administered Monday through Friday by subcutaneous (under the skin) injection. Weekends are periods of nontreatment to allow the pituitary gland's normal feedback mechanisms to maintain equilibrium. A new form of HGH replacement is available as a once-a-month injection.

Thyroid Hormone

Thyroid hormone supplementation involves a dose of 0.5 to 3 grains of triiodothyronine (T3) and thyroxine (T4), most commonly found in the form of Armour Thyroid, an easily available and inexpensive prescription medication. This form of thyroid replacement, as opposed to a synthetic thyroid hormone that provides only T4, is usually the most effective, because it supplies both essential components of the thyroid hormone. Selenium is required to convert T4 to T3. Supplying T4 alone can result in inefficient T3 production because of depleted selenium levels in many individuals. Also, some people have a genetic condition that binds T4 to protein and prevents the successful generation of T3.

Pineal Gland Hormones

Pineal gland hormones are supplemented with melatonin, at 0.3 to 3 mg orally at night before bed. The lower dose is appropriate to aid sleep. At the 3-mg level, melatonin is an antioxidant but rarely a sleep aid. Appropriate melatonin levels have several advantages, which include DNA protection (the antioxidant function), improvement of immune function, regulation of general hormonal release patterns, and, in some cases, improved quality of sleep. People with autoimmune diseases usually should not take supplemental melatonin but can obtain it instead by taking 5-

HTP, the precursor to serotonin, some of which resolves into melatonin. Others can also achieve both improved serotonin and melatonin levels by taking 5-HTP.

Adrenal Hormones

Replacement of the adrenal hormones usually concentrates on DHEA. In women the dose is 5 to 25 mg daily by mouth in the morning. Men can take between 20 and 50 mg daily also by mouth in the morning. Women should keep in mind that most DHEA is converted to testosterone and that an elevated testosterone level can result in elevated 5-DHT, which may cause acne and thinning hair. For this reason, DHEA levels should be monitored closely, especially in women. In men, DHEA is frequently converted to estradiol and can contribute to breast enlargement. The genetic tendency toward breast enlargement is found in a significant number of men. This problem can be controlled by prescribing 7-keto DHEA, a form that is not easily converted into estradiol.

Testosterone replacement can also be provided in the form of transdermal (through the skin) creams, oral supplements, gels, patches, or injections. For women, the recommended transdermal-cream dosage is normally 0.25 to 2.5 mg/mL daily; for men the range is from 25 to 160 mg/mL twice a day.

Estrogen

Hormonal replacement with the triestrogens (estradiol, estriol, and estrone) is recommended for women to mimic the body's natural levels of these hormones. The suggested dose is 1.25 to 5 grams applied to the skin twice daily until symptoms of deficiency (such as hot flashes and vaginal dryness) are eliminated. The ideal approach is to use the lowest dose possible to eliminate symptoms. Progesterone replacement should start with 20 to 200 mg twice a day in the form of a transdermal cream. Progesterone can also be given orally in a dosage of 50 to 250 mg daily (the usual dose is 100 mg) before bedtime. If hormone creams are used, they are applied twice daily, morning and evening, to maintain stable blood levels around the clock. Symptoms of progesterone deficiency—water retention, weight gain, bone loss, anxiety, sleep problems, painful breasts, and shorter menstrual cycles—should also be monitored until subjective improvement is documented.

TECHNOLOGIES, PRESENT AND FUTURE

We stand at the brink of a revolution in anti-aging therapy and technology. Within the next two decades many promising techniques will help us achieve an expanded quality of health and extension of longevity not previously thought possible. Already, breathtaking advances have given us

TIMELINE OF PRESENT AND FUTURE TRENDS IN ANTI-AGING MEDICINE
And What Might Come of It

1999	• Initial stem cell therapy begins • Computerized measuring of biochemical biomarkers of aging
2000	• Telomerase trials begin in humans • 100% of the human genome mapped and sequenced • Legislation enacted to protect Americans against genetic discrimination
2004	• Rudimentary gene chips available to measure changes in "gene expression" as biomarkers of aging • Naked DNA transplants begin
2005	• Test for risk of cancer, diabetes, stroke • Gene therapy for hemophilia, heart disease, some cancers
2010	• DNA chips that analyze a person's genetic makeup and compare it to optimal sequences of genes • Biomarkers of aging now based on gene expression directly
2012	• Medicine tailored to an individual's genetic makeup available to treat diseases, including cancer
2015	• Nanotechnology therapy for aging disorders in humans
2018	• Doctors correct defective genes using combinations of DNA transplants, nanotechnology, and stem cell therapies
2025	• Computer power exceeds human IQ and is used to direct future R&D therapy

the ability to take new anti-aging concepts and turn them into scientific reality. We now have sufficient knowledge to improve the function of our DNA. Anti-aging practice distinguishes itself from conventional medical treatment in that the anti-aging physician is concerned with biomarkers, rather than simply with alleviating specific symptoms of aging. Monitoring biomarkers enables us to evaluate the effects of an individual's anti-aging program. The technologies described here represent attempts to measure and improve the biomarkers of aging.

Gene Banking

What is the optimal level of gene expression throughout life? The answer will differ from one individual to another. One way to answer the question is to establish a baseline biomarker profile based on measurements taken in late adolescence or early adulthood. This allows the anti-aging practitioner to do more than make an educated guess based on the mythical average for a specific biomarker. The ideal would be to perform a complete biomarker survey at or before age thirty to determine an individual's baseline biomarker levels. But even if your thirtieth birthday has long since passed, it isn't too late to find your own current baseline. Without it, you will never know for sure how close you have come to achieving your genetic goals.

The technology of gene banking makes it possible to store and document our genetic profile regardless of our age. As with baseline biomarker assessment, the ideal time to do this is during late adolescence or early

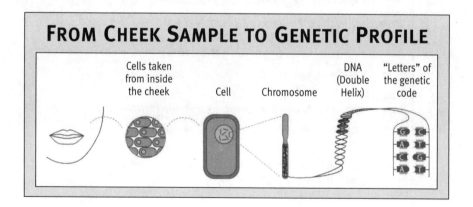

FROM CHEEK SAMPLE TO GENETIC PROFILE

Cells taken from inside the cheek | Cell | Chromosome | DNA (Double Helix) | "Letters" of the genetic code

adulthood. People who wish to pass an anti-aging orientation on to their children should look into gene banking for them, since the next generation is likely to be the first to realize the full benefits of emerging anti-aging technology. Banking our own cells at forty, fifty, sixty, or seventy years of age will still document our present gene expression and will prove useful as new technologies appear. Gene banking is accomplished by taking a small sample of cells from the inside of the cheek and placing them in a deep freeze with liquid nitrogen. These cells can be retrieved at a later date and compared with a current cell sample to assess the health and vitality of the DNA and decide on appropriate improvement strategies. The anti-aging centers listed in Appendix B can assist with gene banking.

Gene Chips and Genomics

While it is fairly easy to document the biomarkers of aging at present, we can only infer from them what is going on at the level of gene expression and guess whether these changes are the result of gene copying or the formation of proteins that the genes make. *Gene chips* will make it possible to realize truly optimal gene expression.

The completion of the Human Genome Project, a major milestone in the history of life on this planet, has now provided the basic code for life as well as disease. We have discovered and can now read the blueprints to design and build a human organism. The appearance of computers with embedded gene chips will make the information about the human genome useful in the anti-aging clinic. This newly deciphered information about our twenty-three pairs of chromosomes will be a primary force in the evolution of our understanding of biomarkers, and will be the focus of a new branch of science called *genomics*.

A gene chip is a flat surface about the size of a thumbnail on which is arranged a specific chain of DNA, containing thousands of DNA sections, called probes. Researchers and, before long, physicians can use the chip to identify particular gene sequences and their variations or mutations. To do this, they take a drop of blood or a tiny DNA sample from the inside of one's cheek. The sample is subjected to a fluorescent dye and applied to the chip. Genes present in the sample will bind with similar genes on the chip, which enables the researcher, using a special kind of microscope, to detect variations and identify possible genetic problems. One such chip is about to be released in the United States. Its purpose is to identify people who have a genetic tendency either to overreact or underreact to standard doses of drugs used to treat disorders such as depression, high blood pressure, and heart disease. The chip analysis will help physicians adjust the dose of a particular drug for a specific patient without the current trial and error that is often necessary. A chip also exists that can scan DNA samples for vulnerability to genetic diseases. Other chips are sure to follow. Eventually there will be a chip that can monitor the expression of genetic sequences involved in the aging process.

Gene chips are also called *DNA chips* or, more generally, *biochips.* The technical term for them is *microarray,* and the process of testing gene patterns of an individual is called *microarray profiling.* Genomics is the field that studies genes using microarrays. In the example of testing for drug resistance or sensitivity described above, the field of study is known as *pharmacogenomics.*

Stem Cells, Therapeutic Cloning, and Regenerative Medicine

The use of bioengineering and cloning of stem cells is being intensely studied in many laboratories around the world. Experiments such as the cloning of Dolly the sheep point to the possibility of differentiating adult DNA, such as that taken from a swab of the inside of one's cheek, into stem cells. Once colonies of stem cells are available, they may allow us to selectively regenerate any component of the aging human body. As the techniques of molecular biology become more sophisticated, cells with specific embryological characteristics will be produced from cells taken from the patient's own body. Body parts will be repaired or replaced using the techniques of human therapeutic cloning.

Eventually many of the surgical and laser technologies presently used to treat the visible effects of aging will be abandoned in favor of actual tissue replacements cloned from our own cells. The use of stem cells should also help to validate the hypothesis that mitochondria are key players in the aging process; this is an area of intense speculation in recent research. Many recent experiments have indicated that aging results in a loss of capacity to repair mitochondrial and nuclear DNA. This loss may be reversed with new mitochondrial elements transplanted from stem cells, introducing new virgin mitochondria into the aging body. If the hypothesis is correct, transplanting one's own stem cells should help to increase ATP production, resulting in the improvement of some of the biomarkers of aging.

More advanced stem cell therapy will also be able to repair organ systems impaired or destroyed with age. Organ-specific anti-aging therapy should be possible within the next decade. Furthermore, stem cell treatment for improved central nervous system function will provide treatment options for the most feared aspect of aging: mental deterioration, age-related memory impairment, and Alzheimer's disease. The anti-aging centers listed in Appendix B can assist with stem cell banking.

Nanotechnology: Molecules as Machines

Shortly after these technologies become mainstream anti-aging therapies, nanotechnology, the ultimate in anti-aging assistance, may be ready for clinical application. Nanotechnology uses molecules as machines to perform specific tasks impossible in any other known way. This technology is superbly suited for making repairs in tiny spaces, such as in arteries, veins, and capillaries. Most likely, surface damage to the skin will be the first area of experimentation. As nanotechnology matures, it is likely to focus on such applications as genetic repair and even remodeling. Biobots, or nanotechnology robots, will be designed to repair and reconfigure DNA, making it possible to reverse DNA damage and inherited genetic defects, as well as to deliver chemotherapy agents to specific cell sites. The application of these technologies will allow for optimal gene expression and repair of either inherited or environmentally caused defects. With this ability, the medical community will be able to push the limits of optimal life and health span to ranges not imagined at present.

ON THE BRINK OF A NEW ANTI-AGING ERA

Over the next five to ten years, anti-aging therapies will undergo a dramatic transformation. The anti-aging clinic of the future will read a patient's genetic sequences and measure gene expression by extracting small samples of DNA, most likely from the white blood cells, to be compared with the optimal age-related gene patterns soon to be defined by the Human Genome Project. This will allow genetic defects to be detected and gene-expression patterns to be monitored early in life. Therapies will be directed at improving the poor expression of specifically inherited genes as well as suboptimal biomarkers. Ultimately, the therapeutic end points will be an increased health span, an improved quality of life, and a slower appearance of age-related diseases. With the use of these new technologies, we will be able to document the effectiveness of anti-aging therapeutics on gene expression that is directly involved in the aging process. One of the most hope-inducing prospects is having the ability to repair telomeres, which seem to determine the end point of cell replacement.

Ten to twenty years from now we can expect anti-aging therapies to involve direct manipulation of genetic sequences within living human beings. Starting with a sample of the individual's DNA, more advanced and highly selective gene chips will focus on the content and expression of the patient's nuclear and mitochondrial DNA. This will allow us to solve the puzzle of cellular energetics (ATP production) and DNA replication. Genomics will be a mature science, providing a more detailed analysis of inherited and environmentally acquired genetic defects. By the 2020s, a vast array of genes will have been analyzed, including those involved in such important processes as hormone production, the transmission of signals within cells, ATP energy production, DNA repair, transcription, translation, and methylation.

The expanding universe of nanotechnology tools devoted to gene manipulation will make it possible to identify defects and ways to correct them, using custom designed, self-directed molecular machines. These unique nanomachines will be designed to carry out intracellular repairs on defective genes according to the information harvested from gene chips. This therapy will be easily administered in the doctor's office of the future. A computerized biomarker profiler, incorporating gene-chip information, will document the results. This approach should make it feasible to extend the span of healthy life and to push beyond the limits of present-day human genetic capacity. The ability to document changes in gene expression and repair of DNA sequences will transform anti-aging therapeutics into a discipline that will be custom-tailored for each individual and each age-related disease process. This technology, coupled with a logarithmic growth of computer intelligence over the next few decades, will allow computers to surpass human intelligence scores and begin to direct future research on aging, as well as age-management treatment protocols. Artificial neural networks, already in use for many nonmedical purposes, will increase our ability to understand complex relationships between different biological systems as we age.

The twenty-first century will usher in a new era of medicine that treats the causes and not the effects of aging, right down to the genetic level. We will be able to control, repair, and re-create our genetic inheritance and, most likely, to direct the quality of our lives and longevity. We will look back on the past few decades and realize that we have progressed from the practice of medicine based on the germ theory of disease to deciphering and enhancing our own genetic makeup and aging codes. We humans, carbon-based life forms, will soon come to realize that we have created a new silicon-based life form called the computer, with an intellectual capacity far beyond our own. Computers will aid us in our quest for enduring health and eternal youth at a speed far beyond our human capability.

While we wait for the arrival of these amazing technologies, we still have the ability to use the information presented in this book to drastically improve the quality of our health and our lives. If we follow the recommendations in these pages, we most likely will be able to maintain our DNA in an optimal state, make full use of our true genetic potential, and be in an optimal place to use some of the amazing technologies soon to arrive.

Ours is the first generation that possesses the capability to reach a state of health and quality of life previously unheard of or imagined in the history of humanity. It is truly an exciting time to be alive.

CHAPTER 8

Quantum Theory: The Final Step in Breaking the Aging Code

Vincent C. Giampapa, M.D., F.A.C.S.

WE ARE ALL QUANTUM FLUCTUATIONS. THAT'S THE ORIGIN OF ALL OF US AND OF EVERYTHING IN THE UNIVERSE.

—John Bahcall, Institute for Advanced Study, Princeton University

Throughout this book we have emphasized the importance of repairing and maintaining your DNA in an optimal state. We have discussed the new horizon technologies designed to add both extended quality and years to our lives. We have described the supplements, nutraceuticals, and nutritional and lifestyle changes that will help you to better use the genes you have inherited. We have shown that the fundamental building block of each of these genes is DNA, and that there is something unique about the DNA in every one of the 100 trillion cells that make up your body. To explore this uniqueness, this final chapter goes beyond medicine to look at discoveries in other scientific disciplines.

The field of quantum physics proposes that all matter is composed of energy that is constantly vibrating at different frequencies. What we see as solid is really composed of subatomic particles in constant motion. Nothing holds still: not the chair on which you sit, not the book you hold in your hands, not the bones in your hands, not even your DNA.

Underlying all of this motion is a ubiquitous force that quantum physics has called zero point energy (ZPE)—energy undetectable by our human senses but present in every square centimeter of air and space. Not only has ZPE been mathematically proven to exist, it has been measured with the latest array of scientific instrumentation. As hard as this is to believe (the idea that your automobile is in motion even when it is parked defies common sense), we cannot reject what science has shown to be true. Yet we hunger for some experiential proof of this transcending, limitless energy, something we can see or feel that provides concrete evidence it exists and makes up all matter.

Perhaps we can find evidence of ZPE's existence in another natural phenomenon, an aspect of nature known as Phi. Also referred to as the Divine Proportion and the Golden Portion, Phi is a mathematical constant found everywhere in nature. The value of Phi is 1.618 . . . (the dots indicate that the decimal number extends to infinity). (Phi is not to be confused with pi, or 3.1416 . . . , the ratio of the circumference of a circle to its diameter.) It is a number that exists everywhere in nature. Phi's ubiquity is beyond mere chance. It can be found in the spirals of the galaxies, the spiral of a chambered nautilus seashell, in the growth patterns of flowers and plants, in the behavior of light and atoms, even in the form of the pentagram (a five-pointed star). Phi is the ratio of the measurement from the tip of any of the Grand Pyramids to the ground, assuming a plumb line could be dropped from inside the pyramid, and from that point to the edge of the structure. Phi defines the dimensions of the Parthenon in Athens. Phi is used in musical composition, and it is found in the human body.

Measure the distance from the tip of your head to the floor, then divide this number by the distance from the floor to your navel, and you get Phi. Measure the distance from your shoulder to the tip of your middle finger, and divide the result by the distance from your elbow to your fingertip. Once again, it's 1.618. Hip to floor divided by knee to floor. Finger joints, toes, spinal divisions, even to the length and width of the DNA molecule itself, all illustrate the ratio of Phi.

Phi is a magical number. We recognize it as evidence of proper proportion even when we are unaware of its existence. But Phi is more than that—it is physical evidence of an underlying energy force. Phi is the hidden order within the chaos we see in our twenty-first century world. When the ancients discovered the Divine Proportion, Phi, they were certain they were observing God's energy flow into the world, giving it the form and substance we know as matter. They saw Phi as the energy blueprint on which all matter is based. Although the existence of this underlying force has been intuited since ancient times, science has measured and scientifically proven its existence only recently.

The hypothesis underlying this chapter—that human DNA acts as a conduit for this all-pervasive energy field—is backed by scientific evidence from many unrelated disciplines. Simply put, DNA acts as the bridge between the world of matter and the world of energy; it controls the flow of ZPE. This control appears to be based on DNA'S three-dimensional shape and structural integrity. DNA's relationship to Phi is compromised and its ability to channel ZPE decreased only if DNA has suffered damage beyond the body's ability to repair it.

Furthermore, recent research has shown that DNA is affected by energy fields generated by the human body itself, as with the electromagnetic fields of the heart and brain. It also appears that emotions themselves may generate energy that alters these electromagnetic fields, affecting the shape of DNA and its ability to transmit its force from the world of energy to the world of matter.

Research at Stanford University has shown that positive emotions (love and compassion) and negative emotions (hate and anger) have opposite effects on the three-dimensional configuration of the DNA molecule. Most significantly, the positive emotions actually create electromagnetic fields that enhance DNA's three-dimensional shape, molding it back toward its ideal state so the flow of ZPE is increased.

Further support for the theory that DNA is a conduit for zero point energy comes from additional information from the discipline of quantum physics. Physicists in the field stunned the world when they suggested that black holes are a source of enormous energy emissions, as opposed to sucking in everything within range and emitting nothing. It was even suggested that black holes might actually form a bridge between parallel universes of energy and matter. Following the ancient adage "As above, so below" (what happens in the micro world of invisible energy happens in the macro world of visible matter), I propose that DNA may be analogous to an extremely small black hole, from which zero point energy finds its way to the physical world through the double helices of DNA's structure.

Support for this notion comes from the fact that it has been proven that DNA acts as a superconductor, transporting electrons down the length of its double helix.

It has also been shown that DNA emits energy in the form of biophotons, which have been measured and scientifically documented. It has been further postulated that DNA's base pairs, and their specific positions and shapes, may act as antennae for specific electromagnetic frequencies, which may determine what proteins or enzymes are produced. These emitted biophotons may actually be the energetic blueprint that directs the physical machinery of DNA to accomplish its specific tasks.

In summary, not only does DNA affect the flow of this universal, ubiquitous, infinite energy source called ZPE, but DNA is also influenced by the electromagnetic energy emitted by the human body itself. As we daily experience the gambit of human emotions, this does not seem so far-fetched. Evidence for the influence of human beings' electromagnetic fields is found in scientific studies showing that energy emitted by human hands can directly affect wound healing, tissue growth, and protein formation.

Perhaps it is no coincidence that throughout recorded history every great religion has emphasized the same message of love: love for God, love for oneself, and love for one's fellow human beings. Love may well be the emotion that gives rise to the energy that restructures and activates DNA and directs the flow of infinite energy into each one of our 100 trillion cells. Perhaps we are just now beginning to understand the basis of mind-body interactions, "miraculous" cures, and "spontaneous" remissions. It may also be that the secret to optimal aging and optimal health has always been encoded within us. It appears that the knowledge given to us by the multitude of scientific and medical disciplines now gives us the means to consciously affect our genetic machinery, our DNA, and make quantum energetic improvements to our health and our longevity.

Food Lists

FOODS THAT RAISE OR LOWER BLOOD pH

It is possible to affect pH levels by adding or omitting certain foods. The items in the following lists are arranged according to their impact on pH, ranging from the greatest impact to the least. (Columns should be read from top to bottom and from left to right.) If you are told your pH is too low (that is, you are too acidic), use these lists to choose alkaline-forming foods and avoid those that are acid-forming until your pH returns to its optimal level.

Alkaline-Forming Foods

GREATEST IMPACT

Figs
Molasses
Olives (green or ripe)
Lima beans
Soy beans
Apricots (dried)
Greens: turnip, beet, dandelion, mustard
Spinach
Raisins
Kale
Swiss chard
Almonds
Parsnips
Beets
Dates
Celery

Rutabaga
Endive
Cantaloupe
Lettuce
Parsley
Watercress
Apricots (fresh)
Potatoes (sweet/white)
Pineapple
Coconut
Pomegranate
Baked beans
Nectarines
Cabbage
Cherries
Sauerkraut
Grapefruit
Tomatoes

Radish
Currants (dried)
Cauliflower
Lemon
String beans
Peaches
Mushrooms
Squash
Watermelon
Grapes
Buttermilk
Whole milk
Millet
Brazil nuts
Buckwheat
Onions
Green peas
LEAST IMPACT

Acid-Forming Foods

GREATEST IMPACT

Egg yolk

Herring

Oysters

Crab

Lobster

Oatmeal

Veal

Sardines

Perch

Salmon

Swordfish

Fish, most

Meats, most

Fowl, most

Liver

Chicken

Pork

Ham (smoked)

Macaroni

Grains, most

Bacon

Lamb

Duck

Egg, whole

Spaghetti

Organ meats

Rice

Bread (wheat/rye)

Haddock

Crackers

Bread (white)

Nuts, most

Egg whites

Corn, dry

Corn meal

Zwieback

Cheese, American

Cheese, natural

Lentils

LEAST IMPACT

LOW-CARBOHYDRATE VEGETABLES AND FRUITS

If you adjust your carbohydrate intake downward to avoid glycation and want to sharply reduce or even eliminate starches, grains, and sweets, you may wonder what carbohydrates you can eat. The following lists answer that question. (Source: *Blood Sugar Blues: Overcoming the Hidden Dangers of Insulin Resistance* by Miryam Ehrlich Williamson. Used with permission.)

Low-Carbohydrate Vegetables

Except where noted, a 3.5 ounce (100 gram) serving contains fewer than 5 grams of carbohydrate.

Alfalfa sprouts	Celery	Onion (1 oz)
Asparagus	Collard greens	Radish
Avocado	Cucumber	Red-leaf chicory
Bamboo sprouts	Dandelion greens	(arugula)
Bean sprouts	Eggplant	Romaine
Beet greens	Endive	Shallot
Bell pepper	Escarole	Spaghetti squash
(sweet green)	Garlic (1 clove)	Spinach
Broccoli	Kale	String beans
Brussels sprouts	Leek	Summer squashes
Cabbage, all kinds	Lettuce, all kinds	Swiss chard
Carrot	Mung bean sprouts	Tomato
Cauliflower	Mushroom	Turnip greens
Celeriac (celery root,	Mustard greens	Watercress
knob celery)	Okra	Zucchini

Low-Carbohydrate Fruits

Even fruits that are relatively low in carbohydrates call forth insulin to handle the sugars they contain. Since one of the goals of low-carbohydrate eating is to require as little insulin as possible, fruit should be considered a special treat, reserved for days on which your carbohydrate intake is especially low. Fruit juices are always too high in sugars to be included in a low-carbohydrate eating plan. The following fruits contain fewer than 10 grams of carbohydrate in a half-cup serving, except where a different quantity is noted.

Apple (sliced)
Apricot (4 oz)
Blackberry
Blueberry
Boysenberry
Cantaloupe
Cherry (sour, sweet,
    10 medium)
Coconut meat (1 oz
    or 1 cup shredded/
    grated, not packed)
Coconut milk

Currant (red, black,
    white)
Elderberry
Gooseberry
Grape (10 medium)
Honeydew melon
Kiwi fruit (1 medium)
Kumquat (1 medium)
Lemon/lime (2-inch
    diameter)
Lemon/lime juice (1 oz)
Mulberry

Orange (sections,
    without membrane)
Peach (1 medium, 4 oz)
Persimmon (American,
    Japanese, 1 medium)
Pineapple (1 oz)
Plum
Raspberry
Strawberry
Tangelo (1 medium)
Tangerine (1 medium)
Watermelon

APPENDIX B

Resources

Every attempt has been made to provide accurate contact information at the time of publication. However, street addresses, telephone numbers, and websites are subject to change. An Internet search engine such as www.google.com can help you if any contact information becomes invalid.

ANTI-AGING CENTERS

Cenegenics Medical Institute
851 Rampart Boulevard
Sir Williams Court Complex,
    Suite 100
Las Vegas, NV 89145
(888) YOUNGER or (866) 953-1530
www.888younger.com

Giampapa Institute
89 Valley Road
Montclair, NJ 07042
(973) 783-6868
Fax: (973) 746-3777 or (973) 746-4385
www.giampapainstitute.com
A full array of anti-aging programs, from the most basic with home testing to those with the most comprehensive testing available. All programs focus on DNA therapy, hormonal replacement, brain health, and growth-hormone replacement therapy.

The Monroe Institute (Mind Body Center)
62 Roberts Mountain Road
Faber, VA 22938
(434) 361-1252
Fax: (434) 361-1237
www.monroeinstitute.org/
    voyagers/voyages

ANTI-AGING AND CANCER-TREATMENT CENTERS

Burzynski Research Institute, Inc.
Stanley R. Burzynski, M.D., Ph.D.
9432 Old Katy Road
Houston, TX 77055
(713) 335-5697
Fax: (713) 335-5699
www.volmed.com

COMPOUNDING PHARMACIES/ANTI-AGING FORMULARIES

International Academy of Compounding Pharmacists (IACP)

P.O. Box 1365
Sugar Land, TX 77487
(281) 933-8400 or (800) 927-4227
Fax: 281-495-0602
iacpinfo@iacprx.org
www.iacprx.org/referral_service/
index.html

DIAGNOSTIC LABORATORIES

Aeron LifeCycles Clinical Laboratory

1933 Davis Street, Suite 310
San Leandro, CA 94577
(510) 729-0375 or (800) 631-7900
Fax: (510) 729-0383
www.aeron.com

American Medical Testing Laboratories (AMTL)

1 Oakwood Boulevard, Suite 130
Hollywood, FL 33020
(954) 923-2990 or (800) 881-AMTL
Fax: (954) 923-2707
www.alcat.com

Douglas Laboratories

600 Boyce Road
Pittsburgh, PA 15205
(412) 494-0122 or (888) 368-4522
Fax: (412) 494-0155
www.douglaslabs.com

Genox Laboratories, Inc.

1414 Key Highway
Baltimore, MD 21230
(800) 810-5450
Fax: (410) 347-7617

Great Smokies Diagnostic Laboratories

63 Zillicoa Street
Asheville, NC 28801
(800) 522-4762
Fax: (828) 252-9303
www.gsdl.com

Immunosciences Labs, Inc.

8730 Wilshire Boulevard,
   Suite 305
Beverly Hills, CA 90211
(800) 950-4686

Kronos Corporate Headquarters

4455 East Camelback Road,
   Suite B-100
Phoenix, Arizona 85018-2843
(877) 667-0007 or (602) 667-0007
Fax: 602-667-7772
www.kronoscompany.com/
science_laboratory.aspx

OptigenexLab
Biomarkers of Aging Panels
750 Lexington Avenue,
    20th Floor
New York, NY 10022
(212) 905-0190 or (866) 678-4469

Quest Diagnostic Labs
One Malcolm Avenue
Teterboro, NJ 07608-1070
(201) 393-5000 or (800) 222-0446
www.questdiagnostics.com

ESTHETIC SURGERY

www.youthfulneck.com
*Website of Plastic Surgery Center
Internationalé for the most advanced
anti-aging surgical procedures
available anywhere. Surgical
procedures are used intimately with
anti-aging therapies to maximize
initial healing and long-term results.*

GENERAL
INFORMATION

www.antiaginginfosite.com

www.worldhealth.net
*Website of the American Academy
of Anti-Aging Medicine.*

http://bioportal.weizmann.ac.il
*Information on each human gene
mapped or sequenced*

PERIODICALS
Anti-Aging Bulletin
IAS Ltd.
Les Autelets
Sark GY9 OSF
Channel Islands, Great Britain

Anti-Aging Medical News
2415 N. Greenview
Chicago, IL 60614

Journal of Anti-Aging Medicine
Mary Ann Liebert, Inc.,
    Publishers
2 Madison Avenue
Larchmont, NY 10538
(914) 834-3100
Fax: (914) 834-3689
www.liebertpub.com

Life Extension Magazine
P.O. Box 229120
Hollywood, FL 33022-9120
(800) 841-5433
www.lef.org

PRODUCTS
Diagnostic Equipment

Bioanalogics, Inc.
7909 S.W. Cirrus Drive,
    Building 27
Beaverton, OR 97008
(800) 327-7953
www.bioanalogics.com

Biological Technologies International, Inc.
P.O. Box 560
Payson, AZ 85547
(928) 474-4181
Fax: (928) 474-1501

Hoch Company
2915 Pebble Drive
Corona Del Mar, CA 92625
(949) 759-8066
Manufacturer of H-Scan system.

Neutraceuticals, Hormones

www.antiaginginfosite.com

www.lef.org

www.optigene-x.com
Source of DNA-repair compounds and high-density nutrient formulas.

www.worldhealth.net

pH Balancing

www.feelgoodfood.com

Skin Care

www.giampapainstitute.com
Physician- and pharmacy-compounded skin-care products for optimal effects.

Cosmetic Skin and Surgery Center
810 Abbott Boulevard .
Fort Lee, NJ 07024
(201) 224-6655
www.cosmeticskin.com

www.nvperriconemd.com
A comprehensive skin-care line of anti-aging products for the face and body.

SEMINARS

American Academy of Anti-Aging Medicine
2415 N. Greenview
Chicago, IL 60614
(773) 528-4333
Fax: (773) 528-5390
www.worldhealthnet.com

The American College for Advancement in Medicine
23121 Verdugo Drive, Suite 204
Laguna Hills, CA 92653
Fax: (949) 455-9679
www.acam.org

Clinical Creations, LLC
Nicholas V. Perricone, M.D., Ltd.
377 Research Parkway
Meriden, CT 06450
(888) 823-7837
Fax: (203) 379-0817
www.clinicalcreations.com

APPENDIX C

Additional Reading

Allan, Christian B., Ph.D., and Wolfgang Lutz, M.D. *Life Without Bread.* Los Angeles, CA: Keats Publishing, 2000.

Anderson, Bob. *Stretching.* Bolinas, CA: Shelter Publications, 1980.

Atkins, Robert C. *Dr. Atkins' New Diet Revolution.* New York, NY: Avon Books, 1992.

Audette, Ray, and Troy Gilchrist. *NeanderThin.* New York, NY: St. Martin's Press, 1999.

Benecke, Mark. *The Dream of Eternal Life: Biomedicine, Aging, and Immortality.* New York, NY: Columbia University Press, 2002.

Coffee, Carole J. *Metabolism.* Madison, CT: Fence Creek Publishing, 1998.

Crawford, Michael, and David Marsh. *Nutrition and Evolution.* New Canaan, CT: Keats Publishing, 1995.

Deutsch, David. *The Fabric of Reality.* New York, NY: Penguin, 1997.

Eades, Michael R., and Mary Dan Eades. *Protein Power.* New York, NY: Bantam Books, 1996.

———. *The Protein Power Life Plan.* New York, NY: Warner Books, 2000.

Evans, W., and I.H. Rosenberg. *Biomarkers: The 10 Keys to Prolonging Vitality.* New York, NY: Fireside, 1991.

Heller, Richard F., and Rachael F. Heller. *The Carbohydrate Addict's Diet.* New York, NY: Penguin, 1991.

———. *Healthy for Life.* New York, NY: Penguin, 1995.

McCullough, Fran. *The Low-Carb Cookbook.* New York, NY: Hyperion, 1997.

McDonald, Lyle. *The Ketogenic Diet.* Kearney, NE: Morris Publishing, 1998.

Mindell, Earl. *Earl Mindell's Food as Medicine.* New York, NY: Fireside, 1994.

———. *Earl Mindell's Vitamin Bible.* New York, NY: Warner Books, 1991.

Netzer, Corinne T. *The Complete Book of Food Counts.* New York, NY: Dell, 1997.

Reaven, Gerald, M.D., and Ami Laws, eds. *Insulin Resistance: The Metabolic Syndrome X.* Totowa, NJ: Humana Press, 1999.

Reaven, Gerald, M.D., Terry Kristen Strom, M.B.A., and Barry Fox, Ph.D. *Syndrome X: Overcoming the Silent Killer That Can Give You a Heart Attack.* New York, NY: Simon & Schuster, 2000.

Sölveborn, Sven-A. *The Book About Stretching.* New York, NY: Japan Publications, 1985.

Williams, Roger J. *Biochemical Individuality.* 1998 ed. New Canaan, CT: Keats Publishing, 1998.

Williamson, Miryam Ehrlich. *Blood Sugar Blues: Overcoming the Hidden Dangers of Insulin Resistance.* New York, NY: Walker & Company, 2001.

Glossary

acetylcholine. A brain hormone associated with memory and thinking.

adenine. One of the four chemical components of DNA.

adenosine diphosphate ribosyl transferase. *See* ADPRT.

adenosine triphosphate. *See* ATP.

ADPRT. An enzyme essential to DNA repair.

advanced glycation end-products. *See* AGEs.

aerobic exercise. Exercise that increases heart rate and respiration.

AGEs. Advanced glycation end-products. Linked protein and glucose molecules that damage tissues and organs.

amino acid. A building block of protein.

anaerobic exercise. Exercise, such as weight lifting, that strengthens muscles. Also called resistive exercise.

androgenic hormones. The male hormones testosterone, androstanediol, androsterone, and androstenedione. Also present in smaller amounts in women.

antineoplaston. A molecular switch that activates tumor-suppressing genes.

apoptosis. The natural process in which cells die and are carried off as waste.

ATP. Adenosine triphosphate. The primary source of cellular energy.

autoimmune response. The immune system's attempt to protect the body from invasion by hostile substances gone awry. Immune cells mistake the body's own cells for invaders.

base pair. Two strands of DNA that make up a chromosome.

biomarker. A measurable chemical substance or physiological value that provides information about a person's health.

BMI. Body mass index, a biomarker that measures a person's weight in relation to height.

body mass index. *See* BMI.

C-peptide. A byproduct of insulin that indicates how much insulin the pancreas is producing.

caloric restriction (CR). The anti-aging strategy of reducing caloric intake by as much as 30 percent to reduce harmful effects of aging. Also caloric restriction with adequate nutrition (CRAN).

carbohydrates. One of the macronutrients. Chains of sugar molecules found in breads, cereals, grains, starches, fruits, and sweets.

catalyst. A compound that causes a chemical reaction without being changed itself.

chromatin layer. The spiral layer that coats chromosomes and protects DNA.

chromosomes. The structures within cells that contain genetic information.

collagen. Connective tissue.

CRAN. Caloric restriction with adequate nutrition. *See* caloric restriction.

cross-linkage. The attachment of glucose molecules to proteins.

cytokine. A kind of immune system cell.

cytoplasm. Fluid found inside cells.

cytosine. One of the four chemical components of DNA.

deoxyribonucleic acid. *See* DNA.

diabetic ketoacidosis. A life-threatening complication of diabetes often confused with ketosis.

DNA. Deoxyribonucleic acid. The receptacle for genetic information that builds cells. Except for identical twins, no two people have identical DNA.

DNA ligase. An enzyme that participates in DNA repair.

DNA polymerase. An enzyme that participates in DNA repair.

double helix. The double-spiral shape formed by twin strands of DNA.

eicosanoids. Chemical messengers that work within cells, often associated with inflammation. Prostaglandins, leukotrienes, and thromboxanes are the three types of eicosanoids.

endonuclease. An enzyme that participates in DNA repair.

enzyme. A chemical compound that acts as a catalyst in causing a chemical reaction.

estrogenic hormones. The female hormones estradiol, estriol, and estrone. Also present in smaller amounts in men.

exonuclease. An enzyme that participates in DNA repair.

FFAs. Free fatty acids. The breakdown products of dietary fat that the body can use for fuel.

5-HTP. 5-hydroxytryptophan, derived from the amino acid tryptophan, turns into serotonin in the brain.

free fatty acids. *See* FFAs.

free radicals. Highly charged atoms and molecules that are missing one electron, making them chemically unstable. Also called reactive oxygen species (ROS).

gene. Component of chromosomes. Genes are arranged in linear fashion along DNA strands.

gene banking. The practice of storing genetic material at very low temperatures for possible future use.

gene chip. A silicon chip that contains genetic information for testing purposes.

genome. The sequence of genes on DNA that spells out an individual's genetic heritage.

genomics. The study of genes using gene chips.

glucagon. One of the hormones secreted by the pancreas, a counterbalance to insulin.

gluconeogenesis. Literally, creating new glucose. The process of drawing glycogen stored in the liver and cells and converting it back into glucose for use as energy.

glucose. Sugar in the form used for energy by the cells.

glycation. The cross-linking of glucose and protein molecules, with harmful effects in terms of aging.

glycemic index of foods. An indicator of how rapidly carbohydrates are absorbed into the bloodstream.

glycogen. Glucose stored in the liver and cells.

guanine. One of the four chemical components of DNA.

gynecomastia. Enlarged breasts in men, caused by an excess of estrogen.

HDL. High-density lipoprotein. The "good" cholesterol, it helps decrease other fats in the blood.

helix. A spiral. DNA takes a spiral shape.

high-density lipoprotein. *See* HDL.

histone. A protective layer of proteins on cellular DNA.

homeostasis. Balance, stability. The body's chief goal.

hormone. A chemical messenger, secreted by a gland.

human genome. *See* genome.

hyperinsulinemia. Excess insulin in the blood, the result of insulin resistance.

hypothalamus. The part of the brain that receives messages from nerves and sends messages to the glands in response.

inflammation. The body's response to infection and injury, normally a part of the healing process. Chronic inflammation is one of the key components of the aging process.

insulin. A pancreatic hormone, ideally in balance with glucagon.

insulin resistance. The result of glycation of insulin molecules, making insulin ineffective in its task of storing glucose in the cells.

ketoacidosis. *See* diabetic ketoacidosis.

ketosis. The state in which fats are burned for energy in the absence of glucose.

LDL. Low-density lipoprotein, the "bad" cholesterol.

leaky gut syndrome. The condition in which food molecules escape through the walls of the digestive tract, robbing the body of nutrients and possibly causing autoimmune diseases.

lipid. A fat molecule.

lipodystrophy. Defective fat metabolism.

lipofuscin. Commonly known as "age spots." Signals an accumulation of oxidized fatty acids and other cellular detritus and a failure of the body to eliminate them.

low-density lipoprotein. *See* LDL.

macronutrients. Proteins, carbohydrates, and fats. The major components of all food.

metabolism. The process of breaking down food and using it for fuel.

methyl group. A molecule consisting of one carbon atom and three hydrogen atoms. *See* methylation.

methylation. The process whereby a methyl group attaches itself to a gene, rendering the gene inactive.

micronutrients. Vitamins, minerals, fatty acids, and amino acids. Components of most foods.

mitochondria. The cell's energy factories. Mitochondria create ATP.

mutation. An error in gene copying and transcription.

nanotechnology. An emerging technology that uses molecules as machines.

neutraceuticals. Medicines made from plants.

NF-κB. Nuclear transcription factor kappa B. A component of intracellular fluid that interferes with DNA repair.

nonenzymatic glycosylation. Glycation.

nuclear transcription factor kappa B. *See* NF-κB.

organelle. Tiny organ within the cells. Mitochondria are organelles.

oxidation. Free-radical damage to cells, with harmful results to genes, cell membranes, and organelles.

oxidative stress. The total effect on the body of damage caused by oxidation.

pH. A measurement indicating relative acidity or alkalinity. A pH of 7.0 is neutral; lower numbers indicate acidity; higher numbers indicate alkalinity.

protein. One of the macronutrients, found mainly in animal products. Also, the main component of cells, of which enzymes are one kind.

reactive oxygen species. *See* ROS.

replication. Reproduction and exact duplication of DNA.

ribonucleic acid. *See* RNA.

RNA. Ribonucleic acid. RNA carries the genetic code from DNA to help synthesize new proteins.

ROS. The latest term for free radicals. *See* free radicals.

serotonin. A brain hormone associated with mood, appetite, and sleep.

single nucleotide polymorphism. *See* SNP.

SNP. The one-tenth of 1 percent of our genes that makes us unique.

stem cell. Cells that carry the genetic code but have not yet differentiated into specialized cells that perform specific functions.

telomerase. An enzyme in some cells that can prolong the life of telomeres.

telomere. The sheathlike structure at the end of a chromosome that maintains the integrity of genes during cell division.

thrifty gene theory. The theory that some people have inherited a gene meant to protect them in times of famine by storing fat when food is plentiful.

thymine. One of the four chemical components of DNA.

transcription. The process in which a base pair, not a single strand of DNA, replicates itself. This process results in RNA.

translation. The process in which a single strand of DNA replicates itself. If the process goes wrong, the result is a mutation.

uracil. One of the four chemical components of RNA. Uracil replaces thymine.

Index